CORE & PATH

IDIOSYNCRATIC

CORE & PATH: IDIOSYNCRATIC

BY PAUL A OMDOLL

ISBN 978-0-9850989-7-1

3rd Edition

CORE & PATH

IDIOSYNCRATIC

By Paul A Omdoll

Special Thanks to the Triune God for the countless hours of support, teaching and guidance that has changed my life and for keeping His promise of blessings through letting go and trusting Him.

Thanks to:

Aaron, Bamidele, Bill, Brian, Chad, Dale, Dan, Janet, Jason, Jennifer, Jon, Kären, Kevin, Mark, Marshall, Martha, Melissa, Michael, Paul, Richard, Ruth Ann, Sarah and Topper.

Thanks to the Networlding Team that brought this book to life.

TABLE OF CONTENTS

PROLOGUE

This book is written for people who have been "taken to the edge" or "hit the wall" in their life. Everyone is moving to an edge in different ways during their whole life. It could be a sudden death of a loved one, losing a job, or being under extreme stress for a significant amount of time. Most people try hard to stay away from the edge. Are you now finding yourself on the other side? At a place where you feel adrift in a big blue ocean with no wind and a broken rudder? Are you at a place with no sense of direction? Do you feel like your life has come to an end, as you know it, as though you've lost control of everything that you were building and controlling? Are you emotionally ready to discover your True Self? If your answer is yes, then this book is a gift to help you discover your "Idiosyncratic" Core and Path, while blessing you with your "Idiosyncratic" Life Purpose.

This book attempts to describe a process for your idiosyncratic restoration that will help you discover your unique Path and develop a deep counter-intuitive rudder. Because the marvelous creation of mankind is that we are unique in relationship to God and His process. You cannot hoist up new eccentrically spiritual sails on your ship of life, if you don't let go and allow God to rebuild a new, stronger and deeper rudder.

The king saw a messenger, a holy one, coming down from heaven saying:

Cut down the tree and destroy it. But leave the stump and the roots in the ground, bound with a band of iron and bronze and surrounded by tender grass. Let him be drenched with the dew of heaven. Let him live with the animals of the field for seven periods of time.

– Daniel 4:23

If you feel that God has cut down your tree and it seems like He is destroying everything you've built, this book is for you. Rest assured God will always leave the stump making your roots grow deeper by banding your life with extra love and support from friends, family and new chosen people that He will bring into your life during this time of restoration.

He will drench you every morning before the sun comes up with His teaching. He will take you through stages of transformation, reconciling you back to Him. This process will transform your life from the inside out. His Divine process planned for you will soften the hardened ground of your heart, so He can plant a seed deep in your heart, then allow evil to help you die to your Ego-self germinating that seed of new life. He will fertilize that seed with love, hope and faith like the perfect gardener. He will nurture that new tender sprout like a perfect father, bringing people at the right time into your life.

id·i·o·syn·crat·ic (id-ee-oh-sin-**krat**-ik) Pertaining to the nature of idiosyncrasy, or something peculiar to an individual: *The healthiest minds are idiosyncratic and unpredictable as they follow the course of self-discovery.*

This book is about discovering your "Idiosyncratic" Core and Path that will change your personal behavioral characteristics, resulting in a change of heart and direction of your life's Path. The way God dealt with me will not be the way He has planned for you. Sometimes God allows our desire for sin to take us to the edge of sanity before we break through our minds wall, like the younger prodigal son. And with others He patiently and gently confronts our sinful Ego-self, even though we hold our ground like the older son in that same story. Because this process is counter-intuitive to the way the world thinks, it will seem that you are reacting highly peculiar to what is happening to you.

Idiosyncratic tendencies are unusual or strange, and not shared by the other people. This is because the mixture of a Divine Spirit and a human spirit in a person's Core has a radical affect in a person's life, resulting in a major change of Path. This makes a person seem peculiar or eccentric to others with a normal world mindset.

After this transformation of the Core you will perceive and react differently to common situations in your life; others will notice a change in your behavior and reaction to situations. This change of heart/mind will give you a freedom from fear and worry over outcomes no one can control anyway. God wants you to follow Him beyond what you can control, beyond where your own strengths and competencies can take you, and beyond what is affirmed or risked by the crowd around you; then you will experience the living God and His power, His wisdom and His love, more than you could have ever imagined. He will call you to follow Him to a place of weakness, where you will risk experiencing the vulnerability of a child so that you might know how strong God is and how much He loves you.

The process in this book will help you discover and restore your Core and Path through a transformational process with profound counter-intuitive insights that were revealed to me over two years of intense daily discovery. This divine process is counter-intuitive to the way you naturally think, but it will resonate as truth deep inside your Core. You might find yourself feeling a little confused in your mind, but feeling comfort and peace in your heart with these concepts.

If you read through this book with an open and honest mind, you will be able to move beyond controlling outcomes that could actually limit transformation. This process has been created to break into YOUR unique Core and Path and no one else's. Idiosyncratic people are really tapped into their own belief systems whether others agree with them or not or even understand their peculiar approach to life. In other words, you are ok being "weird" in your relationship with the world. This book works with your current view of the world without making any judgments.

Once you discover your unique Core and Path you become "inner directed" and you will follow your own heart and mind that God can connect with and guide. You also become more of a keen observer of others and particularly sensitive how other people react to your own idiosyncrasies. What will happen is that you will start to question your common beliefs and expectations for your life that the world and religion has taught you. It will open the door to higher levels of spirituality for your mind and open your True Self to faith and trust in a power greater than yourself. It will redefine what sin is in your mind, what it means to be lost, and what it really means to be saved. You will find a deeper inner life.

You will start to experience what scripture means by "you will be in the world but not of it." People in the world might think you're acting eccentrically. Living a normal conventional life actually becomes difficult once you find your *"idiosyncratic path"* because conventional wisdom will sometimes be in conflict with the counter-intuitive truth. You might even regret that you can't do things the way you used to. It was *easier* then. But you realize you can't go back. This book will change your life in a positive way! Your life will actually become more balanced. You will actually find the peace that your brain will ultimately embrace. Your life will get better each year.

INTRODUCTION

My Story: How my life took me to the edge.

I was at a point in my life where I was becoming frustrated. I was in my fifties and had been working hard enough for thirty years in my current career path and I knew I wanted to do something different. But I couldn't. Why? I did not know what I wanted. That question, for most of us, is the hardest question to answer as we mature.

Did I want to start another company? Start a smaller company? Join a non-profit organization? Or just enjoy my life traveling and spending my money? I kept thinking that *doing* something different would help me find peace at my *Core.* But *doing something* only delays the work needed at all of our *Cores.* I was at this point for over ten years. It's like a married woman who finds herself home alone once her kids are gone saying, "I have to do something for *myself* now." I was living life on what I call the *outer rings.* My wife and I were now home alone and not meeting most of each other's emotional needs. We were friends and for the most part kind to one another, but we were both unhappy at our Core.

We had purchased a second home in Florida, which did help a little. I had a temporary sense of relief of getting away from the pressure. But this, too, was part of God's plan. It's funny that when you have enough money to do the things you want, you don't have enough time. Until you find your True Self at your Core and your chosen Path, these things will not come into alignment in your life. The more you do, the more you have and the more you have to please yourself, you think you will find a place of rest. But it is just the opposite. It seems to get worse. The activity in my life became mind consuming and this left no space for God to get through my mind to my Core.

I was going though a lot of pressure at work at that time. We had acquired a couple of companies that were outside the core competencies of our base business. They were companies that had a lot of commodity type products. Some people kept saying to me that we should not have made these acquisitions. There were all kinds of pressures at work. I personally felt like everyone, from all directions, was giving me the look of judgment that screamed "Boy, you made a big mistake this time!" It felt like the right thing to do at the time but most of the feedback around me was negative as we uncovered what we had truly acquired with the first acquisition.

But I felt strongly that if we could take this company with its commoditized products and turn them into value-added products with a strong trusted brand, it would pay back. As our innovative products were integrated in with these high volume products and we added differentiated features to these commoditized products, we would have a more powerful mix. But the negative feedback from others kept getting in the way and delayed the integration that was needed for the distribution channel, market and operational synergies.

Additionally, I was under a lot of pressure at home with my son trying to find his way in life. It seemed that every choice he made was making his life harder. I have a daughter who is a clinical psychologist who tries very hard to do the right things every day and takes full responsibility for her life. It's a proven fact that a person's strengths are also their weakness, and my children have different strengths and weaknesses.

If opportunities don't unfold fast enough for my son, he moves on to the next opportunity. He is truly a deeply bright young man and if he learns to plan and articulate his direction, my son will get the results that he so desperately desires. As my only son, I just did not know what to do. It is always tempting to throw money at any problem to make it go away, but in my heart I knew it would make it worse for him. I needed to let go and allow each of them to build their own financial base before I could start to support them. Giving either of them money too soon could cause more problems in our relationship.

Helping your children grow stronger and healthier with money at the right time is like applying fertilizer. If they are supplying the water and have enough sunshine getting to their Core each day, money can be helpful. Adding fertilizer in the wrong season of their life will only cause more damage to their True Self. Arguing on the phone with my son—that disconnection, misalignment and feeling of failure as his father—was so frustrating along with everything else going on at that time, and contributed to pushing me to the edge.

That year, we upgraded our timeshare condo in Cabo San Lucas, Mexico where we would finally have room for our whole family, including the grandchildren. We had been going to Cabo over the Christmas/New Year holidays for years. It doesn't take long to figure out that kids will go almost anywhere when you pay the way. We were all getting excited to go to Cabo and enjoy the new condo. We were going to be able to spend two weeks together as a family in a place we enjoyed with less pressure from our busy lives.

But what I did not know is that my wife was already planning to leave me. That same December we were getting new furniture for our home in Wisconsin. I can now only assume that her intentions were to get all the improvements done that we should have done over the past ten years, in preparation for the divorce settlement.

One evening before we left for vacation, however, I started getting sick. I felt better the next day, but the stress was still intense. What was happening in my body was that my adrenaline levels were building in my blood stream. It was constricting all my arteries. I understand now this was happening because of the sustained high stress levels. And because I was recovering from a 24-hour flu, my blood was now getting thicker, entering a hyper-coagulated state.

As I was coming home from work the next day, I experienced a sharp deep pain in the right side of my neck. I thought it was just one of those stingers that I had felt before from moving the wrong way, but my body felt strangely weak for a few minutes, so I was a little concerned. I had no sense that anything was really wrong. I even made a phone call to a good friend for the rest of my drive home.

I was focused on getting home to meet a truck driver who was delivering our new furniture that night. When I got home 15 minutes later, I stopped in my driveway to walk over and get our mail from the mailbox, like I had done a thousand times before. But when I got out of the car, I couldn't stand up without feeling like I was going to fall over. I used the side of the car as support to get back in and sit down. I felt okay again so I decided to drive the car up to the house.

As I was driving up the driveway my eyesight was starting to get blurry. When I got the car into the garage and got out, I found myself feeling as though the left side of me was three times heavier than my right. I was like a drunken sailor on a steep angled sailing ship.

I finally got in the house using my hands to stay off the walls. Everything became blurry. My mind was screaming, "What's happening to me?" I was confused and disorientated. I thought I needed to get upstairs to get some aspirin in me, but had further difficulty getting up the stairs, holding myself away from the walls again. When I made it to the upstairs bathroom I could no longer stand up so while on my knees in front of the vanity, I looked frantically for aspirin, but ended up only finding Tylenol before I had to lie on the floor to stop the disorientating dizziness.

I managed to call a friend from work with my cell phone. I guess my speech was so bad by then that she didn't know whom I was. She thought it was a very old man trying to reach someone. She was worried he needed help and her husband took the phone and looked at the caller ID. Then he knew it was me. They ran out the door with their six-month old baby to come to my rescue.

I called my wife next and told her that I did not feel well. My words were getting more slurred by the minute. I told her, "Look, I am not going to be able to answer the door to let the furniture delivery guy into the house. I can't move from this spot!" My wife asked if she should call 911, which I responded with a frantic "yes"! The driveway soon filled up with police cars and fire trucks. Even the furniture delivery semi truck was next to the ambulance.

At first everyone thought it was that there was a natural gas leak in the house, which is why the fire trucks were there. I kept trying to explain to the paramedics that it wasn't anything that was going on in the house. I grabbed the young paramedic by the shirt and pulled him closer, looked into his eyes and said, "Listen kid, it's not a gas leak, I was losing control before I entered the house. Trust me; it's something with my neck!"

What was strange was I did not have any of the usual symptoms of a stroke. No reduction of strength in my hands or feet, loss of feeling on the surface of my skin. But my vision and speech were being dramatically affected. That's because I wasn't having a typical stroke in my cerebral cortex; it was a stroke in my cerebellum. That is the smaller part of the brain that controls your involuntary muscles like your heart and lungs.

When I got to the hospital they had to do a scan of my brain to see if I was having a brain aneurysm before they gave me anything to thin my blood. While we were waiting for the results, they sat me up to check my vital signs. That's when the second infarction happened and I could feel the left hand side of my body getting cold.

The next morning the neurologist came to my hospital room to see me after examining my record. He believed that a small tear in one of the vertebral arteries in my neck caused a place of turbulence spinning two tiny balls of clotted blood, which then flowed directly into my cerebellum.

If it wouldn't have been for the adrenaline coating like a varnish around those clots, they would have dissolved only blocking blood flow in my cerebellum for a short time. If that were the case I wouldn't have had a major stroke. But because those two clots blocked fresh blood flow to two areas of my cerebellum, it resulted in brain tissue dying behind the blockage. This affected my equilibrium and the ability to sense temperature on the left side of my body.

Interestingly enough, this incident was the first of three major changes in my life that actually helped me hit the wall and allowed God to start the transformation process of my Core. This exposed the right path that was chosen for me from before I was born. The neurologist assigned to me at the hospital said, "If one of these clots would have floated up into an area an eighth of an inch from where it did—it would have stopped your lung function and you would have died in 15 minutes. No one could have saved you. God must have a plan for you."

I learned years later that I actually have a Lupus antibody in my blood. This is not connected to Lupus at all other than the first patient they discovered Lupus in also had this antibody so they thought there was a connection. Today it only carries the name. They are now finding out that this antibody was formed in one of my ancestors years ago when they were exposed to something. It was formed and passed on through genetics over generations.

The doctor said that they have now found out that people who have these antibodies are at a much higher risk of strokes in their forties and fifties. So the doctor highly recommended my children and siblings get tested. I started thinking that because of this "close call" I should do something different with my life. But it was about *doing* something different again, thinking that would fix my Core. That first major intervention of God was the stroke—which I am assuming was planned from my birth (aka the genetics pre-disposed in me)—softened the ground of my heart hardened by life.

The next thing that happened, or should I say didn't happen, was that my wife decided to delay divorcing me. She chose to be there for me during the rehabilitation from my stroke. What would people say if she left me now in this condition? She also thought that perhaps because I hit the activity wall with this stroke, it would change me to be a better person. Well, it didn't. My behavior got worse. I reacted to everything at the same level of intensity during my recovery. I actually became short-fused. My neurologist and my daughter, a clinical psychologist, told me that it wasn't that unusual. Any type of rebalancing of your chemical system can result in you becoming short-fused but people see you as being unreasonable with your reactions to issues. The first few months I would have regular daily bouts of anger over little issues.

What's strange is that during that summer, after six months of recovery, I had a unique and stage-setting visit by two business associates, a husband and wife team from Chicago involved in World Vision. They were there for both the major changes in our business relationship and their personal caring relationship with me.

They also shared their pictures of Zambia in Africa where they had been involved for over seven years setting up what World Vision calls "Area Development Projects" (ADP's). These initiatives involve 15 years of work that, at the end, the Zambian government would take over responsibility and the support services, making these gifts of personal resources sustainable.

They told me later that they felt directed to ask my wife and me to go to Africa with them for some reason they didn't understand.

I had been promising my wife of thirty plus years that I would take her to Africa someday on a Safari, so when this opportunity came our way just after my stroke, we both felt we should do it for different reasons. She had always given to World Vision children for years and she always wanted to go to Africa to see the animals. She let me know, "I want to go with or without you!"

I thought to myself that after this stroke that could have ended my life so abruptly, that I better take her before I couldn't. I was also fortunate enough that my partner in business supported us going. That gift has turned out to be a life-changing event for both of us. This trip was what they called a Vision Trip, not a missionary trip. Most of the time we spent in ceremonies turning major projects like schools, medical clinics, student dorm facilities and fresh water wells over to the Zambian government to maintain and develop. Putting a well in a village is the cornerstone of any developing community. It changes everything for the people of that village.

I asked one of the translators assigned to us from the local World Vision team, "What did you do for water before this new well was put in the village?" He said, "I actually grew up in this village. I was the one chosen to get the water every day as I was the strongest in the family." I asked, "How long did it take you to get water?" He responded with, "It was a two-hour walk to the closest river, twice a day, once in the morning and then again in the afternoon." I couldn't believe his answer. That was eight hours a day just getting water for his family. I said, "Now, that you have this new fresh water well, think of all the things you can do to improve your village."

"Yes, it changes everything," he said.

I realized that this single well now enabled all the productive people in the village to really improve the health and lives for hundreds of Zambians now and in the future. Think about it. This fresh water that would change all their lives forever has been sitting right under their feet for hundreds of years. Once you get your head around it that this fresh water is the foundation of life in so many ways, you have to do something. Now, because of the well, children are not dying of simple diseases and they don't keep getting sick from bacteria filled water. Between the water and AIDS I am amazed that anyone is still alive in Africa today. You come away understanding how this one small investment changes an African village forever.

I've created a website for this initiative called www.hearts4zambia.org. The site links to organizations that are approved by Zambia to help their people. I have found out that there are some organizations that you can give to for Zambia that the resources never get to the people, for many reasons.

We traveled to Africa in the summer of 2008 after making the decision in 2007. It took one full year of planning and preparation to go to Africa with World Vision Chicago. When we were there,

I took over one thousand pictures during those two weeks. I think I did this because I felt more comfortable hiding behind the camera. I felt empathy, but it was hard for me to get engaged personally with the children, because I didn't know how to help them so I didn't want to get too attached. I tend to approach things from the top down—like a business owner, before I get emotionally involved in a project. My ex-wife, on the other hand, was more about leading from the heart. She was there for more about connecting with the children and made a powerful impact each day with the people in every community.

At the final evening dinner before we left Africa, the leader of the Vision trip (one of the Vice Presidents of World Vision, and now the CEO of Living Water International) shared with us that there are one of three things that tend to happen to people after they experience what we experienced here in Africa.

One is that nothing major changes in your life when you get back home, but you see things from a totally different perspective even though your life does not take a major change. Others go back home and find their lives hold no real meaning compared to their experience in Africa. You don't feel your job is worth it anymore and there's little value or impact in your life which you feel is wasting away in whatever current situation you're in. The third thing that can happen to people is that a seed is planted in your heart and you don't even know it. You plan on going back to live your normal self-controlled life, but what you don't know is that seed that God has planted in your Core will start growing in you and that seed will completely transform your life.

So the stroke had softened the hardened ground of my heart so that God could plant the seed in my heart during our Africa trip. I used to think I couldn't afford to give of myself unless it would benefit me in some way. Yet there were definite seeds planted in Africa by people who, on the surface, I didn't feel could help me in any way back home in my complicated life. I was very much wrong.

Instead, those people turned out to be a life-changing gift to me. They helped me "hit the wall." They helped me *"breakthrough"* my mind's wall of paradigms and get to my True Self hidden deep in my core.

Two weeks after we returned, my wife connected with someone she went to high school with. Shortly after that she came to me and said that she now had two loves pulling at her heart—the children in Africa and this friend from back in high school.

In a matter of weeks my wife of thirty-five years was telling me she did not love me anymore and that if I truly loved her I would be happy for her and let her go so she could be with him. My heart broke into pieces. My mind went into shock. I felt as if a doctor was telling me I only had a limited time to live. My life was coming to an end the way I knew it. That was when my life hit the wall for the third time. This is when the seeds from Africa had to die in me to germinate and sprout new life through God's merciful restoration plan. However, because the ground was softened and the seeds were able to take root in my life-hardened heart, my ex-wife's rejection helped me let go of my self-controlled life.

I believe that if the first two events hadn't happened, I would have just become more narcissistic and self absorbed after my divorce. But instead God's perfect plan of restoration started.

I know in my heart that if I had not had the stroke, the seeds of Africa would not have taken root and then if my wife had not divorced me, I would not have been able to break through my mind's wall. It wasn't just the end of the marriage. It was the end of the dream of trying to do the right things for myself to be happy and content with my life. My concern is for my ex-wife and the difficult path she has embarked on. She believes that God told her to divorce me and marry this other man. She told me that God was punishing me by taking away my beautiful wife and my money, and giving it to this friend, who was a man of God. She went on hoping and praying that God would bless the two of them for divorcing their current spouses and being together. I believe, just like me, she needs to face herself, instead of thinking her happiness will come from others.

I had to "leave my cave." Everything I had built there was coming to an end. All that work suddenly had no value. I had to walk away from everything I had built. In my own narcissistic way, that's what I was experiencing. I moved into an apartment. I was at a place I did not want to be. I had never rented a place to live up to this point in my life. This was the time of facing the consequences of my self-serving choices all these years.

God spoke to my heart directly when this was all happening to me. I sensed from Him that if I didn't let go of my whole life and give it back to Him, He would take away more things I valued and that I thought I had control over in my life. This is the order I felt God was going to use until I gave in to Him: My wife, my money, my children, my business skills and my health.

I felt He was in the process of having my wife taken from me at the same time the economy started to hit the wall. It seemed as my thirty-five years of work to build a strong secure financial nest egg was all falling apart. Remember I had just had a stroke, so I knew God could take my health at anytime He chose.

I was getting ready to fly down to Naples, Florida by myself because this time my wife had decided that she was not going with me. I found it interesting that I had booked this trip down for a week over six months before, just hoping that we could get way to enjoy our second home. It was that week that God chose to really get directly involved in my life.

That's when I started writing. Strangely, three people that week told me directly, by stopping the conversation, to tell me that I should start writing down my experiences. In fact, that night before I left for Florida I was having dinner with one of my good friends that had become a Christian just over the last few years and I started disclosing what was happening in my life. He informed me that he felt that God was telling him that I should start writing this stuff down. I disagreed at that point. I had never written anything in my life and I was not about to start now.

I would rather "build" or "start" something instead of document what had happened in the past. I knew he had good intentions, but I questioned if he was getting a message for me from the God of all creation!

As I was waking up the next morning I distinctly heard God speak to my inner mind, urging me to write my thoughts down. Reluctantly, I went to get a piece of paper and pen. I wrote a little.

After a couple of days in Naples I called one of my colleagues, an engineer by trade, a mature Christian friend, who said to me, "I think you should start documenting what is happening." His comment started to stick. The next morning as I was praying I said to God, "I don't trust my own brain and I don't trust most Christian brains. I don't want to make stuff up. In order to prevent this, I need You to confirm it three times with three different external sources so I know it is really You, God. I had two people tell me to document God's intervention in my life."

After I returned to Wisconsin I met with yet a third person that told me the same thing. The third person added that "I should not just write it down, but document it electronically, converting it to a word document." I was reluctant because it seemed at the time to be a lot of extra work.

But other messages that came that week in Naples were beyond just documentation. Three other people in one day that had never met each other said the exact same thing to me—exactly the same words—one person at lunch, one person on the phone late that afternoon and the third person that night at dinner. The exact words were, "You can't go back." This was in reference to the change occurring at my Core.

This was the beginning of a journey that I didn't ask for, but God had planned for me before I was born. Jesus appeared to my mother in the hospital at the foot of her bed and told her to name me Paul after the Apostle Paul. The Spirit revealed to me, through a spiritual counselor that He brought into my life, that I would be going through seven stages of an orderly transformation process. I had lost control of my life at that time, so I figured—I'll go with the flow.

These were the seven stages of my restoration process:

1. Intervention
2. Healing
3. Restoration
4. Renewing of Heart and Mind
5. Walking in Humble Spiritual Growth
6. Walking in Truth & Wisdom
7. Rest, Release, Refocus, Reset & Restore

Here are excerpts from my personal journal that the Spirit had instructed me to document by confirming it three times through three different people. As you will see below, God intervened in my life every day for one solid month. I suspect God knew He had to be really direct with me to get through this hard German/ Norwegian brain of mine.

My Intervention (Sept. 20th – Oct. 20th 2008)

God had decided to move in my life, and this is the recording of His loving intervention and the beginning of His healing and restoration in my life, starting Sept. 20, 2008 but first I will explain what ultimately pushed me in this stage.

On Sept 17th I chose to confront my wife with the knowledge of her rebuilding a relationship with an old friend – now current love – from back in high school. He is a Messianic Rabbi/Minister and a parole officer in Texas. I didn't know at that time that God had his hand deep in that situation as well.

Hearing about this was a stab in the heart that pushed me from the shore of my own life into His River of Living Water (God's will) from those years ago I was baptized in and had been drinking from, swimming in, and washing myself when ever I chose. His Holy Spirit would call me too, while always returning to the shore protecting my sinful and disobedient life from His truth for the last thirty-five years. I was being carried down His River for the first week, with my head held under water by His hand, having my nights slow down and my days speed up.

This is a detailed record of what the Holy Spirit took me through as God chose to intervene in my life to save me from myself.

Important dates in 2008:

- *I am pushed into a River of Truth by my wife's rejection. Sept. 17th*
- *God starts the reconciliation process in Chicago. Sept. 20th*
- *God has me go to His altar with a Christian friend as my witness. Oct. 8th*
- *God has me confess my sins to Him and my wife, asking for forgiveness. Oct. 11th*
- *God is concluding my intense intervention phase. Oct. 25th*
- *He is now starting my healing and restoration phases. Oct. 26th*

Note the perfect timing and alignment around the Day of Atonement:

- *Exactly 3 <u>days</u> between Sept. 17th and Sept. 20th*
- *Exactly 3 <u>weeks</u> between Sept. 17th and Oct. 8th*
- *Exactly 3 <u>days</u> between Oct. 8th and Oct. 11th*
- *Exactly 3 <u>weeks</u> between Sept. 20th and Oct. 11th*

- *Oct. 8th is the Jewish Calendar Day of Atonement*
- *Oct. 11th is the Jewish Biblical Day of Atonement*

Friday, Sept. 19th

My wife has had enough with my self-absorbed life, and feels that God is calling her to do "God's Will" without me holding her back. She gave me a book of Jesus' life written from scripture in chronological order as a story. This really helped me get started looking back into "God's Will" for my life. On Friday morning I woke early to pray, cry and read. When my wife woke up, I reached over to take her hand. The moment I touched her hand the Holy Spirit came rushing over me. I was so ashamed of my relationships with both my wife and God. I turned my head away in shame and started weeping uncontrollably for about two minutes. After that I started to pray for God to start dealing with me to change this wretched man that I had become.

Saturday, Sept. 20th

The first day of my restoration process started when I went to the Bible to find the scripture verse my wife had on her cell phone as the caller ID name for her friend from high school. It was his initials and 10:12. I looked in every book of the Bible, starting with Genesis until I got to Mark in the New Testament and it was like hitting a wall of truth.

Mark 10:12 reads:

"And if a woman divorces her husband and marries someone else, she commits adultery."

When I told her of my discovery, she told me that I should hold onto that verse. I was confused why she would use that verse on her cell phone while reopening her past high school relationship and closing down our marriage.

That same day we drove down to Chicago to spend the weekend together and visit a female pastor of a church in downtown Chicago, keeping our promise we made in Africa to a new friend. She was with our World Vision group that traveled to Africa the last two weeks of June 2008. That afternoon my wife and I went shopping on Michigan Avenue. As we were walking south on the east side of Michigan Ave, we decided to cross to the west side of the street.

As we crossed over the street and got to the corner, we realized the sidewalk was blocked for construction. As we turned around to join the other people waiting to cross back over to the east side, a man standing on the corner by the new building under construction was holding up a Christian tract in the air.

He yelled out, "Do any of you know who this is?" It was a bad print job of Jesus hanging on the cross in black and red ink, showing his blood being shed on the cross. He then yelled out, *"Raise your hand if you're not ashamed of Jesus."*

My hand went up instantly without even thinking about what kind of a nut this was on the corner. My wife then followed my lead and raised her hand from out of the group. He pointed at us and yelled out, "Because you were not ashamed in public of

Jesus, He will not be ashamed of you in front of the Father." He then said, "I tell you this: You are going to Heaven!" The light changed and we walked back over with the group to the other side of the street and I felt like we had been in the presence of an angelic being.

That night we went to a new restaurant in the new Trump building on the river. After a pleasant dinner we stopped at the hotel's bar for a drink. It was noisy and busy. We then started to throw our conversation in snippets back and forth to each other over the noise. It started out happy and pleasant, but then turned direct and nasty as we started to be honest with our hurt feelings about our past 35 years. We then stopped and agreed to be nice to each other for the rest of the weekend.

Well, that only lasted for the first third of the walk back to the hotel where we were staying. It was a beautiful summer night in Chicago for a walk, but I could tell my wife had become extremely distant, so I started to become very direct with my feelings, to the point of talking in her face abusively. She responded and our conversation got deeper, exposing all our hurt feelings and blaming each other for everything we could dig up from our thirty-five years of marriage. This continued until we arrived at the front of our hotel. This was the convention tower of the Hyatt Hotel along the river, so the activity was very low that time of night. We sat down on a bench in front of the hotel to continue our direct unloading of our long, unhappy relationship. It got downright ugly.

A nice man in his late forties walked up to us and interrupted our verbal battle, to ask us if this was the stop for the shuttle bus heading to the casino. We reacted with anger letting him know we had no idea and gave a look that clearly meant "leave us alone so we can finish our fight to the death."

He then walked away about 50 feet from us as we got back into verbally stabbing each other with the frustration of our past relationship, focusing our rage to cut as deep as we could to hurt each other's feelings. The man walked back towards us and sat down right next to my wife.

Interestingly enough, there were no more than a few inches showing on the bench next to her. He pushed himself onto the bench next to her that forced her to move towards me to the point where I had to get up to make room for both of them. He just sat there looking forward without uttering a word. I asked my wife to get up and go with me up to our room. She was fuming and resisting the temptation to tell this man off for being so rude, but she didn't.

I now believe that he might have been the second angel sent to intervene in our lives that day. As we were getting ready for bed, God had me get the Gideon Bible from the hotel room, directing me to some verses that I never knew were in the Bible. He was speaking to me through the Word "He is tired of my sinful walk and if I don't change now, He will throw me out of his Kingdom."

God has been a loving Father all my life and I have pushed His grace as far as I could. He said, "If you don't start bearing good fruit; I will cut you down like a dead tree." I felt like I was on my way to hell! I was shocked that my loving Father, that had told me my whole life how much He loves me, was now telling me the same thing my wife had been telling me. They were both throwing in the towel and were walking away from me. That was a heavy way to go to sleep that night!

At about 3:30 AM the Holy Spirit woke me up in the hotel room. I sat up and started praying in the dark with my wife quietly sleeping next to me. He then did a Scrooge type thing, showing me the relationship between my son and I, pointing out how he is living in self-denial and self-absorbed narcissism. Showing me how sad it makes a father.

I love my son, but I couldn't and can't do anything to help him until he starts making better choices and faces himself at the Core. But God revealed to me that He felt this same way about me. He also showed me that my sins of my bad temper, ego, and lust of the flesh were genetic. My father and brother had the same issues as my son and myself. If I wanted to help him, I had to allow God to deal with these sins in myself first and as a result, God could help me break these generational sins in our family.

By then the light of the morning was starting to gently light the room. God had me make two lists of names that he wanted me to contact, one list was people I had hurt with my temper, ego and selfish needs. And the other list was people that he wanted me to share what was happening to me for some reason. At that point my wife woke up slowly and quietly next to me. God had me ask her to pray for me.

I thought she would say no way, but instead she reached over lovingly and took my hand to pray for me. She prayed the most calm, humble, loving, caring, compassionate prayer for me that I have ever heard. There were no hidden agendas of condemning me or subtly making a point, for the entire five-minute prayer. At that point the Holy Spirit poured over me. From that moment on early that Sunday morning, God started his four-week intervention with me, non-stop day and night. *One solid month!*

That morning we left the hotel to head to the church. On the way to the car, we quipped that God would probably have something in the sermon that would match up to what we were going through in our relationship. "Let's see how much," we both said. When the service started we realized that the title for the new series of sermons ahead was starting that very day. It was named "get-GOD, get-Messy, get-Good" boldly over the cover of the bulletin for the service.

When the reading from scripture took place, a very sophisticated looking older couple went to the front of the church. Each had their own podium. They started out each reading scripture to us softly and lovingly. The husband had scriptures about God's forgiveness with His believers and hers were about God wanting us to face the sins in our lives, showing the contrast between

His unconditional love for us and our shameful disobedient human behavior.

As they got into verses that got more direct, they started raising their voices and began reading the verses at each other as arrows back and forth, similar to our behavior the night before. They were moving their podiums away from each other and not caring about the rest of us in the audience. They were consumed with making their points to each other. That she should learn to forgive or God won't forgive her. And he should be honest with himself and his sin or God would not forgive him. My wife and I shared the same thought: we wondered if they were trying to make fun of the personal struggles we were having with each other.

The pastor (our friend from the Africa trip) got up and started reminiscing about her trip to Africa and had the two of us stand up to be recognized as a loving Christian couple that went with her which was very humbling! She proceeded with the sermon, explaining how when God would move in a big way on this earth, He would always allow things to get messy and confusing, just before He brought about a powerful change in the current situation to align things with His will and plan of reconciliation and restoration. After a nice lunch with the pastor and her family, we drove back to Wisconsin.

Monday – Friday, Sept. 22nd – 26th

Every night was long and difficult. I woke up many times less than an hour after going to bed or by 1:30 a.m. in the morning to pray and read something from the Bible looking for answers; piece by piece I was peeling back the layers of my deep ego filled sinful self. This continued all week, with every night going by slow and the days going fast.

I started working through the people on the list at work that I had hurt with my rude temper outbursts or condescending comments. God had me tell them about certain episodes of God intervening during my weekend in Chicago, and that they were on my contact list. I started with my boss, business associates and old friends.

My wife left on Thursday night that next week to drive her mother and sister up to where her mother grew up as a child, which she had done many times before. This gave us both the space we needed from each other after a heavy weekend. That night, I had dinner with a good friend that is living a new intense relationship with Christ. As I was telling him what was going on including looking for some advice from God, my friend told me to start writing things down that God is revealing to me. I said to him very directly, "*I don't write things down.* But if this is a word from God, ask God again while you're driving home and if He tells you again; call me on your cell and I will consider it."

He never called.

The next morning when the Holy Spirit woke me up again, God spoke to my heart to start writing everything down. I called my friend that morning and told him that God just confirmed it directly to me. Then God gave me Psalm 103 as my idiosyncratic chapter. At this point I didn't understand this would be like a syllabus for the course that God the teacher was going to cover over the next year.

LET ALL THAT I AM PRAISE THE LORD!

I have included Psalm 103 in the Appendix just incase you are reading this book without a Bible with you. This is the main reason I have inserted scripture within the book. Please read other versions of the same scriptures I have used, so God can use them to speak to you about your Idiosyncratic Core and Path.

PSALM 103

Saturday, Sept. 27th

I was flying down to our 2nd home in Naples, Florida by myself and God had put it on my heart to start working on the contact lists. First He wanted me to talk to my wife's Christian sister. So during the limo ride from the airport, I called my wife's cell phone and asked her if I could talk to her sister. She said she was in another room at the hotel in Escanaba, Michigan and she would tell her my desire but wouldn't promise she would talk to me. God then told her sister before my wife could tell her about my call, that God had a chapter for me to read and I was suppose to figure out what three verses God wanted me to hear. As I was flying down to Florida, God put on my heart what He wanted me to say to her sister. First that God is moving and He is dealing with many core issues in my life and I believe He is calling me to do something for Him in the future. But, before I can move forward on any of this, I needed to take the time to set things right with people I have hurt; and she was one on that list!

God had me tell her that I should confirm her faith in God was real. Also, that her faith was new and fresh and mine was old & stale. I was also sorry for being so rude to her when she was trying to help me with fresh advice from God's Word. I also told her about what God had shown me about Aaron, and how I have a similar relationship with God. He also told me I should listen for God's voice through her from now on. Then I thanked her for caring about my sole like she does.

Sunday, Sept. 28th

God had me up again at 5:30 a.m. praying and reading all morning the book *The Life of Jesus* my wife had given me. I went for lunch on my Harley and found a Christian Family Bookstore to buy a Bible. I couldn't decide what version to buy, so I bought two versions. Now God could start talking to me directly from His scriptures again. God revealed to me that morning that He is working in my wife's life at the same time, and that she has been holding things in her heart for years that needed to be removed before God could use her in His work. It became very clear to me that my wife will not comfort me during this time of God dealing with my sin.

I can't hide from God anymore behind my wife's good works.

God is giving me one more chance to start bearing good fruit, or He is going to cut me down like a dead tree, as He so clearly pointed out to me in the Bible. Doing His will is not hard or confusing. It's simple and clear: just obey when the Spirit talks to your heart. Just when you think He is going to ask you to do something difficult, He asks you to do something simple in faith. *(2 Kings 5:1-19)*

God's kindness brings us to repentance, not His law!

I thank God for my Christian friend from Milwaukee. He called me every day and night to check on me, sharing words and scriptures from the Lord for me each day, until my wife arrived in Naples. That Sunday night I called my daughter and told her what I thought God was doing in my life and would be sending her a letter telling her how I felt about our relationship at that point. She said that her pastor at their church just gave a sermon that day. He told his church he was leaving to do other work for God and it was very much the same thing I was telling her that God was calling me to do. She said, "The two of you needed to talk ASAP" to which I agreed to enthusiastically.

Monday, Sept. 29th

This was an interesting day with three completely different individuals.

The morning started by God waking me up early again for Prayer and reading. God took me through the conversion of Saul to Paul, showing me my link with Paul in the New Testament and with David in the Old Testament. At about 8:30 a.m. EST I was moved to call my wife.

I called her and shared a few things that I had thought God was telling me. She said I needed to listen more than talk and that God is calling out his people for His work. She told me this multiple times over the last week. My friend from Milwaukee called within seconds of hanging up from my wife. One of the first things he said was God had told him that I needed to listen more than talk today in addition to how I can't go back to my life of sin and walking in my own will. He shared that he feels God is calling him to challenge Christians to follow His will, and that God is calling out His church from all religions.

My day started with my good friend from Naples who came over with his Harley to go for a needed long ride. I was looking forward to a normal worldly day with a break from God's pressure. Boy was I wrong. We stopped for a beachside lunch up in Fort Myers Beach. We sat looking out at the gulf then I started telling my friend what God was doing in my life, step by step. He told me his story of alcoholism and how his life went all the way to the bottom, to the point of almost taking his own life one day. He enrolled in Alcoholics Anonymous (AA) and he told me God was taking me through the exact same process of the 12 steps to recovery and he recited them at the table from memory. He turned to me looking straight in to my eyes with a very stern face and said, "You can't go back ever again." He was not talking about getting drunk in sin, but that I could never take a taste again, or it would be much worse the next time.

Later that afternoon I was looking forward to a little time away from God's hand on my neck, and a normal business dinner. A business associate was picking me up around 6 p.m. and I had a little time to kill. I looked at my list of other people to contact, and saw the name of an old friend that had just moved back from Hawaii to Atlanta, that I hadn't seen for years. I thought about taking his name off the list because he was a friend that was as narcissistic as I was. But, God moved me to call him instead. He answered the phone and we exchanged greetings. I started telling him what God was doing in my life. When I finished, I just calmly asked him if there was anything he wanted to tell me. The phone went silent first and I heard weeping and crying on the other end of the phone so hard he couldn't talk, although he kept trying.

This went on for several minutes. I kept reassuring him to not rush it. Finally he was able to compose himself enough to start telling me something that blew me away. He began to let me know how he really felt about me. When he saw me calling, he wasn't going to answer it but let it go to voice mail. But thank God he answered. He proceeded to tell me he didn't think he would ever tell me this, but that he couldn't stand my "all about me" narcissistic attitude that had developed over the past years. He didn't want to be my friend anymore by that point but he said he recognized things were changing for the better, and he was glad that this was all happening to restore our friendship.

The next day or two I got an email from him saying he was really glad that I had called. He apologized for getting so weird, but it was almost like he had no control over his emotions. He guessed someone really wanted him to tell me something they thought I needed to hear. He also went on in his e-mail about how shook up he was but that I should feel free to contact him anytime if I ever needed an ear.

After that I called my wife who knows this friend well, and told her what happened. She told me I had better keep my mouth shut at dinner and I didn't need to be talking to everybody about what was going on in my life. I agreed with her and was looking forward to a nice, non-heart wrenching business dinner. Again I was wrong.

The businessperson I was going to dinner with came to my home to pick me up. As we were driving out of the gated community, he turns to me and says, "Well what are we going to talk about tonight? Business, personal stuff or what is going on with our wives?" I couldn't believe it. I said, "I don't think you want to hear what is going on in my life, it is too crazy," which he responded, "Fine. Then I will tell you about mine." I responded, "I think I understand why God told me this morning to listen more than talk today." He appreciated that and proceeded to tell me about his current situation with his wife over the last few months. He said his life was a living hell the past few weeks.

He had been struggling between leaving his wife or staying and helping her through her issues. He shared that he read the Bible every morning to help him be a better person in everything he does because he tries hard to do the right things everyday. He thanked me for listening to his issues and said he had told me more that night than he had told his best friends.

He asked me what was going on with my life. After his disclosure, I couldn't hold back any longer. I told him some of the things that God was doing in my life and that I thought God wanted me to share. He said that tonight at dinner I was already a changed man from the Paul that he used to know and my old person was an egomaniac, which was the only thing about me he didn't like. The truth hurts, doesn't it? Even though I knew it was the truth. I guess you just never want to accept things like that about yourself. Your ego doesn't like being attacked. He also said that he believed that if I had died from my stroke, I would have gone to hell. Just like my other friend did, he looked straight into my eyes with a firm expression and said, "You know **you can't go back.**" We finished paying our bill and left for home.

On the way back to our homes, we found humor in how we didn't speak one word of business all night long. We agreed there would be another time. When we pulled into my driveway he didn't say a word, and I didn't feel I should just get out of his car. He looked over and thanked me for the best night of his life. "I know this might sound weird, but I think I'm supposed to pray for you," I said. "Would you?" he asked. "No one has ever done that before for me." So I put my hand on his shoulder and prayed for him. God humbled his heart and spoke to him that night. WOW, what a day I exclaimed to myself.

Wednesday, Oct. 1st

Next on the list to make phone calls were my two sisters. I called the one closest to my age first. She listened quietly and said she would pray for me. I had asked her if she had anything I needed to hear. She said "No, not at this time." My other sister was next. This took place just before my wife was going to arrive in Naples that night.

Actually, my call took place outside the quiet small airport just before midnight, where it is normally full of activity all day. When I asked for feedback from her, my sister gave me three pieces of advice: Actions speak louder than words, faith without works is dead, and I need to spend more time with my mother. I understood and thanked her. At that point I went into the airport and met my wife. We went to bed as soon as we got to our Naples home.

Thursday, Oct. 2nd

I woke up an hour later, just like I had been doing every night back home in Wisconsin. It seems like the best time for God to get through to my heart and mind, without my own internal voices blocking Him, was from 1 a.m. to about 3 a.m. in the morning. Below is what He taught me that night, just in time for the next few days I was going to spend with my detaching wife.

God directed me to read Proverbs to prepare me for communicating with my wife over the next few months.

Proverbs 15

A gentle answer deflects anger, but harsh words make tempers flare.

Gentle words are a tree of life; a deceitful tongue crushes the spirit.

The Lord detests the way of the wicked, but He loves those who pursue Godliness.

Whoever abandons the right path will be severely disciplined, whoever hates correction will die.

A wise person is hungry for knowledge and truth, while the fool feeds on trash.

A hot-tempered person starts fights; a cool-tempered person stops them.

It's wonderful to say the right thing at the right time.

"For I know the plans I have for you," says the Lord. "They are plans for good and not for disaster, to give you a future and a hope."

Jeremiah 29:11

CONTROLLING THE TONGUE

1 *Dear brothers and sisters, not many of you should become teachers in the church, for we who teach will be judged more strictly.*

2 *Indeed, we all make many mistakes. For if we could control our tongues, we would be perfect and could also control ourselves in every other way.*

3 *We can make a large horse go wherever we want by means of a small bit in its mouth.*

4 *And a small rudder makes a huge ship turn wherever the pilot chooses to go, even though the winds are strong.*

5 *In the same way, the tongue is a small thing that makes grand speeches. But a tiny spark can set a great forest on fire.*

6 *And the tongue is a flame of fire. It is a whole world of wickedness, corrupting your entire body. It can set your whole life on fire, for it is set on fire by hell itself.*

James 3:1-6

Truthful words stand the test of time; but lies are soon exposed.

Proverbs 12:19

Friday, Oct. 3rd

My wife woke up early while I was up and I shared some of what God is showing me. Remember God had revealed to me that she would be blinded from His work in me and will not comfort me during this process of Core cleaning and intervention. She thinks I'm too dramatic, and I shouldn't become so emotional about what God is doing in my life right now "because it won't last! Also, God is not done talking to me through non-Christians."

Tuesday, Oct. 7th

I asked my wife if it was okay to talk to her new friend, the Rabbi and ask him if he could explain the Day of Atonement and the meaning of being a Christian today. She agreed. So I humbled myself and made the call. He first explained October 8th was the calendar day, but Saturday October 11th was the Biblical Day of Atonement. And if I am a born again Christian then I am a Jew in God's eyes. That's why he thought God was preparing me for the Day of Atonement. And if he was my Rabbi, he would tell me to be totally honest with God and bring my sins to leave them on God's altar, and I should fast on the Day of Atonement.

Then he told me the story of the two goats: one was sacrificed and the other let go in a field and set free. He also said that both Jesus and Barabbas had the same first name (Yeshua) and they sacrificed the innocent goat and let the guilty one go, fulfilling the Old Testament scriptures. I shared the four things God has been putting on my heart to bring to Him at His altar: my temper, my ego, my sins against God and my wife, and my marriage. He then offered to be my Rabbi if I wanted. I thanked him and I said I would pray about it.

Wednesday, Oct. 8th

My wife told me this morning as we got ready for work that God is pushing her to move and do something. She said that her grandchildren, her old friend and Africa were still pulling at her heart. Our home in Wisconsin and myself were holding her back from what was pulling at her heartstrings. I find it somewhat confusing that God was trying to break up a marriage covenant, but I was in no position to argue the point. I was excited to meet an old Christian friend of mine for dinner that I have total trust in his love and care for me, including God's will for my life. I had made this dinner date with him when I was back in Florida. This was before I knew that same night was the start of the calendar Day of Atonement. We met at 6:30 p.m. at sunset. This was the first person I was to tell what had been happening to me in complete detail over the last three weeks. I couldn't cry at all that night telling the story. I guess I had dried up all of my tears although my friend broke into tears many times during the long dinner. He then said God wants to use this detail to bless other people in the future. Also, God directed my Christian friend to share *Philippians 1:3-11* with me as a word from the Lord.

3 *Every time I think of you, I give thanks to my God.*

4 *Whenever I pray, I make my requests for all of you with joy,*

5 *for you have been my partners in spreading the Good News*
about Christ from the time you first heard it until now.

6 *And I am certain that God, who began the good work*
within you, will continue his work until it is finally finished
on the day when Christ Jesus returns.

7 *So it is right that I should feel as I do about all of you, for*
you have a special place in my heart. You share with me
the special favor of God, both in my imprisonment and in
defending and confirming the truth of the Good News.

8 *God knows how much I love you and long for you with the*
tender compassion of Christ Jesus.

9 *I pray that your love will overflow more and more, and that*
you will keep on growing in knowledge and understanding.

10 *For I want you to understand what really matters, so that*
you may live pure and blameless lives until the day of
Christ's return.

11 *May you always be filled with the fruit of your salvation—*
the righteous character produced in your life by Jesus
Christ—for this will bring much glory and praise to God.

We left the restaurant and got into my car to talk for a while and the night ended when he prayed for me. He was my witness that I put my list of sins on the altar before God. After the heavy time at God's altar, he became very direct with his voice and told me that God was telling him that I should document everything that is happening to me in detail, because God was going to use it later. I was with him from 6:30 till midnight that night. It was a wonderful night of release and comfort for me since the beginning of my journey.

Thursday, Oct. 9th

The first young Christian friend I told you about that had been checking on me everyday, sent me the scripture verse for a Bible study he invited me to that evening. It was 1st Timothy 1:3-7. I found this quite interesting, just after my wife's old friend came back into our lives and offered to be my Rabbi while he was pursuing my wife. This is just how God works. My friend made a mistake when he told me the verse to study. The Bible verse for the study was 2nd Timothy 1:3-7. But God wanted me to read this instead.

Warnings against False Teachings

3 When I left for Macedonia, I urged you to stay there in Ephesus and stop those whose teaching is contrary to the truth.

4 Don't let them waste their time in endless discussion of myths and spiritual pedigrees. These things only lead to meaningless speculations, which don't help people live a life of faith in God.

5 The purpose of my instruction is that all believers would be filled with love that comes from a pure heart, a clear conscience, and genuine faith.

6 But some people have missed this whole point. They have turned away from these things and spend their time in meaningless discussions.

7 They want to be known as teachers of the Law of Moses, but they don't know what they are talking about, even though they speak so confidently.

1st Timothy 1:3-7

Saturday, Oct. 11th (Biblical Day of Atonement)

Early at 5:30 am, I woke up again. This time God put it on my heart to confess all my sins over the last 35 years to my wife, and asked if she could forgive me. She said she had forgiven me years ago, but it didn't change the fact that she had lost all her feelings for me. I said I understood and thanked her for letting me bring my sins to God's altar with her as my witness. It was still dark. I felt like I should get up and put some clothes on to go outside. I didn't know why, but I felt that I should go for a walk with God. I had never done this before, so I didn't know what to expect. As I walked down our long driveway in the dark and as I got half way down, I started weeping uncontrollably.

The Holy Spirit came over me. I walked down to the end of our driveway and up the dark street. I thought God wanted me to keep walking up the street but as soon as I got to the center of our cul-de-sac I dropped to my knees and started thanking him for loving me so much. I looked up and the sky was full of stars without a cloud in sight. I felt like God was looking down at me and directing my every step, just like I had a GPS system in me *(God's Positioning System).*

I got up to start walking back to my driveway and before I took just two steps, a car came driving down the hill towards me. If I would have been there on my knees in the middle of the street just seconds more, it would have been very awkward between the driver of that car and I.

God has had perfect timing in my life over the last three weeks, so there could be no doubt He was directing my every step and every moment. I thought it was going to be a squad car, but it was the paper delivery. I walked back up the driveway to the back deck of my home and sat down on one of the chairs. At that moment, God spoke to my heart directly to let me know I didn't need this Rabbi as a teacher of the truth, and that Jesus wanted to be my only Rabbi. Then God asked, wasn't He teaching me enough each day? He does have a sense of humor and perfect timing. I finally went back to sleep.

> 26 *I am writing these things to warn you about those who want to lead you astray.*
>
> 27 *But you have received the Holy Spirit, and he lives within you, so you don't need anyone to teach you what is true. For the Spirit teaches you everything you need to know, and what He teaches is true—it is not a lie. So just as He has taught you, remain in fellowship with Christ.*
>
> 1 John 2:26-27

I left the following morning to meet another old friend that had become a Christian. He had invited me, when I had talked to him from Florida, to go to his Bible study on Saturday morning and meet the person that brought him to the Lord. He was the leader of this group of about 50 older men from over 30 denominations. They were seasoned in the Lord, humbled by the truth of their own sin and God's grace in their lives. The Bible study leader was a coach and counselor for ministers of God and churches. I met with my friend for breakfast after the Bible study but I was still fasting for the Day of Atonement, so he ate and I talked. He was the other person in my life that God wanted me to go hash out, in detail, what God was doing with me.

We went back to his place of work and sat outside where we could soak up the beautiful sun's rays that morning while he patiently listened to my story. He said the same thing as the two other Christian friends. Take all my hand written notes and put them into an electronic format for safekeeping and for future use. They all said that God is telling them to tell me to do this, so I can go back to it later. I had no idea at that time that I would ever write a book. It was the last thing I had ever desired to do in my life. And I've wanted a lot of things.

Sunday, Oct. 12th

I awoke from a dream, or vision, this morning. I say this because I don't know for sure what it was. God had netted me from the rough sea of this world and I have been flopping on the floor of His boat for three weeks like a fish struggling to breathe. My wife is also in the boat just sitting back and watching the whole thing. It feels like God has now put me in a bucket of water in His boat so I could breathe and to start His restoration process. I am to let go and trust God for both my wife and me 100%.

Monday, Oct. 13th

Time will reveal God's work in me, and expose what is false in me. I will find healing and answers when I minister to others. I must seek His will for me every morning for the rest of my life. I can never go back to my old life.

Be patient with God's work in others surrounding me, and in myself. Don't try and make things happen faster than God wants to move. He is a God of order and process. I must learn to trust His perfect timing in all things. Then the Spirit directed me to Exodus 34 like he had done so many times before by having me just open the bible and start reading.

"YAHWAH – THE LORD"

6 *The LORD passed in front of Moses, calling out, "Yahweh! The LORD! The God of compassion and mercy! I am slow to anger and filled with unfailing love and faithfulness.*

7 *I lavish unfailing love to a thousand generations. I forgive iniquity, rebellion, and sin. But I do not excuse the guilty. I lay the sins of the parents upon their children and grandchildren; the entire family is affected—even children in the third and fourth generations."*

Exodus 34:6&7

This is a very powerful part of the Bible, because these are God's direct Words to His creation from His Core.

Friday, Oct. 17th

God woke me up at 5 a.m. I prayed that God would bring His Spirit over me. It wouldn't come for the first time in 4 weeks, no matter how hard I tried. It had always come over me within seconds of me spiritually looking up to Him from my True Self. Then God said to me, "Go to my written Word." I picked up my Bible and the little book light because it was still dark in my bedroom. I prayed for God to direct me to what he wanted me to read. I opened the Bible like other times over the last four weeks and started reading scripture just like before. I opened it and my eyes locked into PSALMS 103. The Holy Spirit spoke to me that this was going to be my gift from God as an outline for my idiosyncratic teaching through this amazing journey.

Then God spoke to my heart that I needed to confront my sinful ego-self.

Seven Deadly Sins

1. *Short Temper*
2. *Ego Centric Attitude*
3. *Sexual Behavior*
4. *Unfaithfulness to God's Covenants*
5. *Controlling Behavior*
6. *Rebellious Attitude*
7. *Verbally Abusive Outbursts*

God put it on my heart to come before him every day and give up control over these human sinful parts to Him, showing Him that I loved Him in return for saving me from myself.

"Everything rides on Hope, Faith and Love" I recalled.

I am no longer totally in control of my own life. God was starting the long hard work of renewing my Idiosyncratic Core.

Saturday, Oct. 18th Letter to my wife

I had decided to send a letter to my wife because a highly respected female Christian pastor from a church in my area told me that I needed to do what I thought I needed to do to save my marriage. If I didn't, I would regret it for the rest of my life, believing in my mind later that I could have done something to save it. My letter expressed that I was sorry for all these years of suffering I had put her through and how now she was suffering more while I was going through God's restoration process. I did let her know she had every right to reject my appeal for another chance and that I would respect whatever decision she made.

Sunday, Oct. 19th

God revealed to me this morning that I have no foundation started at all yet. I guess this is a slower process than I thought. I am so used to fixing things fast but that's just another one of my human ego-driven parts that work against God's will. God has shown me that during this last month, He has cleared the land, cleaned out the rocks, dug the trenches, and poured the footing on solid ground. Only now can He start to build a strong foundation for a true relationship with me.

God is taking myself from me for others.

Monday, Oct. 20th

While driving to work today I was listening to a Christian radio station and they told a story of a little girl that wanted a little fake pearl necklace from a local store. Her mother told her if she really wanted it, she should save her money until she had the two dollars to buy it some day. Her grandmother gave her money on her birthday, so she now had enough to buy it. She felt so big and proud that she wore it everyday. Her father who loved her very much, and read to her every night, came up to her bedside to read a story and asked her if she loved her new necklace. She said yes, she loves it so much. Then her father asked her if she loved it more than him, and she replied of course not. Then he asked her if she would give him the necklace? She slowly presented it to him.

At that moment my mind went back to a day in Africa when I encountered a small boy about four years old during the trip to Zambia. I had bought some candy from a World Vision micro-financed store in one of the remote development areas. It was smaller than many closets here in the US.

I started handing the candy out to all the children in that area of the village. When I had two pieces of candy left in my hand, I told the kids they were all gone. The children scattered. There was one little boy over by another building just standing and holding his hands up by his face. I walked over to this shy boy and I thought he hadn't gotten any candy. I knelt down in front of him and asked him if he got any candy. He slowly opened his hands and he had one small piece of candy he was saving for later. I put out my hand and asked him if I could have that piece of candy.

He looked into my eyes and he slowly put the piece in my hand. I then put the other two pieces of candy into his open hand. He grinned from ear to ear and ran off very happy.

Just then God said to me: "Will you let your wife go and give her back to me?"

I instantly started crying and accepted God's request. This was extremely painful emotionally to let her go and trust God totally with my future. At lunch I realized I had to *"let go"* of everything in my life, to start this seemingly appointed healing process of my Core: My Ego-self, my wife, my children, my money, my things, my skills and even His Kingdom work at this time. I felt like Abraham did when God asked him to sacrifice his only son, but there was no other sacrifice provided.

> *Bring all the tithes into the storehouse so there will be enough food in my Temple. "If you do," says the Lord of Heaven's Armies. "I will open up the windows of Heaven for you. I will pour out a blessing so great you won't have enough room to take it in! Try it! Put me to the test! Your crops will be abundant, for I will guard them from insects and disease. Your grapes will not fall from the vine before they are ripe." Says the Lord!*
>
> Malachi 3:10-12

Monday Night, Oct. 20th

I was blessed to have the World Vision VP that was on our trip to Africa drive up from Chicago to have dinner with me and stay overnight at my home. At dinner I started to tell him what had been happening to me. He told me his story about what happened to him years ago, when God intervened for a solid month in his life to save him from his rebelliousness.

He informed me that I should prepare for God to start pulling His covering protection away so the teaching process could start. I told him it had been exactly 30 days of heavy intervention by God...until today. He responded that he wasn't saying it would be 30 days for me also which I understood.

You grow through failures in your life. I was now learning the hard way. I truly see clearer now because of those times of weakness and being humbled.

Our guest woke up early the next morning and made some notes for me he thought God wanted me to know.

Here is what he said:

> *God is truly moving in my life.*
>
> *He will restore all good things in my life.*
>
> *God's engaging me to restore my relationships (wife, children and friends)*
>
> *God will use me someday in His Kingdom work.*
>
> *I should not jump into any one thing at this time.*
>
> *I should dabble gently in different opportunities of God's work.*

While he was driving back to Chicago, he called me and said he just wanted me to know that my wife had told him that God was telling her to leave me. He said: God never tells anyone to leave his or her marriage, but he didn't confront my ex-wife at that time. His observation was—we were using God's will to hide behind—and we both needed to take responsibility for our decisions going forward.

That day my intense intervention from God's heavy hand came to an end.

Our Core and our Path were chosen for us before we took our first breath. It's not about starting a new path. It's not about ***creating*** the person you want to be or what your spouse or parents wanted you to be. You can't start ***doing*** the right things to ***be*** the right person. It's about ***discovering*** your True Self so you can ***be*** the right person at your Core. Then you will start ***doing*** the right things without much effort. The more you try to change your Core by controlling the people and outcomes around you, the more you become unhappy with your life. It's not about managing the activities in your life that surround your Core, it's about letting go and letting God do His perfect work in your Core, bringing out your True Self.

This book is about *discovering your True Self at your Core and revealing your Right Path.* I am capitalizing these foundational terms so they stand out for you. You will eventually discover during this process what really lies at *your* Core, not the adapted person you have become conforming to the world around you. This book will take a counter-intuitive look at your beliefs, what drives your choices and the relationship you have with God.

Understanding how to work with God, not for Him is the key

It's amazing as you go through life long enough to look back over your past, seeing how you worked so hard trying to make your life turn out the way you thought it should, trying to control everything that could happen to you. You naturally want to control the day, the year, next year and your future years, all with the intent to get the outcomes we think make us happy or even content.

As you get older you start making major decisions for the future. Then life happens and things don't turn out the way you planned. You have "directed" your path by trying to ***do*** the right things and control all the outcomes. You ask yourself over and over,

"Am I ***doing*** the right things?" It happens with relationships, with careers, with your self-development.

You finally get to the point that you become so frustrated, that you feel you have to "***do***" something about it, or you at least get to the point of saying, "Someday, I have to make a change."

But you don't. You may say things like, "by the time I turn a certain age, I will do "this" or "that."

Trying to control outcomes of major milestones in your life will leave you without much success!

In essence you are living the life that you don't want and are trying to change the Path you feel stuck on.

There are also emotional needs embedded in us that every person desires at their Core. When you don't get those needs met by God or your life partner, you will seek to get them met by others in the world around you—co-workers, your children, even strangers.

The level of importance to you of each of these emotional needs change with any major eventful change in your life: you get married, have children, go through a spiritual awakening, etc. When your life becomes so fragmented that you are seeking to get your emotional needs met by others, rather than allowing God to address them at your Core, you get closer to the wall in your mind.

The truth is—you have to *be* the right person at your Core to start doing the right things in your life, not the other way around. The more you try to *fix* your own Core, the further you get away from God's grace. Our basic emotional needs and human desires actually drive us to the *edge.*

Our natural human evil desires and God's given Laws are beautifully designed to work together to take us to *the edge or wall* so we might let go of our *Ego-self* and turn to His grace for help. Some people get there quickly. Most get there slowly over many years. But, almost everyone gets to the wall at some point in his or her life, even if it is on his or her deathbed. Some people might stand at *the wall* until they take their own lives if they don't break through.

Some people seek Eastern religions that teach self-help healing of the Core. Some pursue any of the multitudes of self-help processes to grab another rope when they are at the end of theirs, just to help them back away from the edge. Others hit the wall hard enough with a major loss in their lives that they break through the wall of their own minds with all their deep-rooted paradigms, exposing their Core to God's merciful light. The more you are self-absorbed and being unfaithful to God at your Core, you seem to move faster to *the wall.* You don't think you have been unfaithful to yourself, but you have. Your deceptive Ego-self has been holding down your True Self for years. God desires for His crown of creation, that all humans die to their naturally developed Ego-self, so their Core can be transformed through Christ blending with your True Self at your Core. You then become a child of Adonai.

Adonai – Hebrew Name for God

Adonai is the plural of Adon, **meaning** "Lord, Lord, LORD, master, or owner" (the word Adon derives from a Ugaritic word **meaning** "lord" or "father")

You believe in your mind you are not worthy. If you have had a spiritual awakening in your past and you know you have held some cards back from God for self-preservation. You need to completely die to your Ego-self at your Core. It's amazing how many Christians I have talked to who have sheepishly said, "You know, I did hold some things back when I came to the Lord also."

Those things you hold back at your conversion will take you to the edge later in life. God knows when you are holding something back, anything, from your spiritual heavenly Father.

"Life's best pathways for the most marvelous transformations almost always come as a surprise. The untransformed cannot invent their own path to transformation. It is rather the Creator who has the power to carve the path and the grace to mercifully light the way that he has planned for us."

Our job is to just walk in that light.

What is really interesting about this light issue is that each of us has a searchlight. We are using it to try and find our way. Some go to coaches, counselors or even psychics to get a larger searchlight to help find their way. But to really see the light it's just the opposite. You have to turn your searchlight off and trust God to open your heart to see the dimly lit path He has planned for you. You might ask why God would make this important path "dimly lit." It's because He gave us the gift of choice and He wants us to choose His Path over our own. That's why we need to take our own path to the edge of disappointment before we are willing to shut off our personal searchlight.

Everything in this book that has been revealed to me seems to be counter-intuitive to the why we naturally think or have been taught, i.e. "you have to actually lose your life to gain it" or "God blesses those who are poor in spirit for the Kingdom of Heaven is theirs." You will hear more concepts like this throughout this book, but I will help you follow this new Path and exploration of your spiritual Core.

Most people don't trust God enough to turn off their own searchlight. Most people want to see before they believe, and understand before they take a step of so-called faith. They spend a lot of time trying to figure out where God wants them to go. That's why so many people do nothing or do evil things in the name of God. For example, The Crusades were done in the name of God, which is the main reason some in the Muslim religion want revenge with evil-ego driven Christianity.

My Idiosyncratic Journey

As I look back over the past few years, I can now see that every major and minor event that had happened in my life and the people around me had an orderly purpose in my transformation. I am sure as you look back you will see that God had His hand in your past also. One of the critical events for me was buying a second home in Naples. I felt that nothing was changing in my life.

I felt trapped in my own self-centered life. I had hoped that if I bought a home in Naples, FL and started to spend more time there with my family, maybe my life would start to change for the better. This decision was self-driven to try and find some personal reward for pushing the rock all those years. Now just a few years later I live in Naples full time, God has blessed me with a wonderful partner and through her kindness, she is showing me how simple faith and kindness can become a deep rudder in my life. You might be wondering why I am telling you about this relationship. Well it's because God revealed to me while I was in Naples the summer of 2009 that He will restore my marriage covenant with Him after He transforms my heart and mind to be a good life partner for someone in the future. God loves to restore and reconcile. Here is what was revealed to me back in 2008.

God seems to be revealing to me that the wife He will bring back into my life to restore my marriage covenant will love God and will respect the work that God has planned for me from before I was born. She will also have a spirit of peace and comfort that will help guide me through challenging times. She will help correct my course, not buy showing me where I am wrong, but through kindness, love and mercy I will be brought to repentance as God continues to make me more like His Son Jesus Christ. Perfecting my faith and using me through my weaknesses to show His glory to help others that are called to follow Him.

I now know God cares about every detail in my life. I also believe that if God is not intervening in your life, you will not find this book as relevant. But if He is then I am here to tell you that you are not losing your mind. You are finding your True Self and Spiritual Core. There is a link between what you are feeling and thinking with what God has planned for you. This information of God's restoration process will be your foundation for release and trust in Him and His orderly process during the next seven chapters.

This is God's process that He has used from the beginning of time. When you read the Old Testament, you will see this over and over again. God is a *gentle*, *firm* and *just* Father. He will nudge you in subtle ways—through people, through messages and through outcomes that happen to you—all to help direct you to your personal idiosyncratic plan of transformation.

This process is beyond human control. Therefore it is beyond your control. This is part of His divine process of calling us back to Him. I now can see this is happening to many other people that God has brought into my life these past few years.

God is asking me to use all the skills I have gained in the world to offer them back to Him for His glory, so that when our sin and the Law take us to the edge, this counter-intuitive process of restoration can be less confusing for our heart and mind.

He is so complex and so perfect that when He does intervene in a human's life, He never does it for a single purpose. It always has hundreds and hundreds of repercussions affecting others, just like sin does. It is no longer a temporal connection, but we now have a spiritual connection directly with the God of all creation. *How wonderful is that?*

God is the Creator of all things and in total control of all outcomes. He is the only one who knows the future because He is not restricted by time. Even Jesus said He did not know the future when He was physically among us. For God to connect with us He needed to create a spiritual bridge because we were born in sin with a dead spirit and spiritually disconnected from Him.

That is why God had to act on His love by coming into His creation in the form of the man called Jesus, the perfect sacrifice. When we read the book of Job, we see that although Job did everything right, he still had problems with his relationship with God. He cried out, "If I only had an advocate!" because Job needed a direct link with God. God created this need for an advocate, a Messiah, from the beginning of time as a way to give of Himself as Emmanuel (God with us). Jesus said I have to go so that I can come back through the Holy Spirit. Then He could become the communication ID with Faith as the password.

That separation from God happened through *one man* Adam, also *one man* Christ (God with us) is the restoration path for all creation. In this way God can be true to His Core of Love, Grace, Truth and Light!

Once we are connected we are able to receive His Spirit into our True Self, then we can communicate directly with God without needing a spiritual translator. The only thing that hinders or blocks that direct connection with God is our minds. That's why we need to break through our minds wall and get to the other side of self to hear His subtle voice. It's critical that we keep that connection open with a little one-on-one time with God each morning.

Back to my story

During the summer of 2010 after my divorce, while I was visiting my grandchildren in Denver, this same Spirit of God woke me early before sunrise. I sat up quickly saying to God, "I don't know why you are so involved in my life like this. It is like I am your only son." God was so intense in my life I thought I was actually losing my mind sometimes. I didn't know this was a good thing at that time. I didn't even think about what I was saying and how wrong it was to be comparing myself to Jesus. Then at that moment I understood the feeling that motivated God's fatherly attention in me. The same way I feel about my children. God said back to me,

> *"Paul Omdoll alone has no value to communicate with me. It is only because you have my Son within you that you are getting my attention."*

When you allow the Spirit of God into your Core, He becomes one with your spirit and that choice allows God to start caring for you as your perfect Father. You can't get that direct Fatherly help unless you have His ID and password in your spiritual Core. The Holy Spirit is there to help God communicate back and forth with you.

God LOVES to tell His children the future, to build solid trust and faith in Him. The Bible is filled with accounts showing how God loves to reveal the future to those He had chosen. God says this is one attribute that separates Him from all other Gods. Only He knows the future. If He didn't reveal it to some of His creation, knowing it alone would have no value.

It's like knowing now that we are in the end times of this age. I know in my heart and mind we are in that season of His plan. The Bible is filled with God revealing what is going to happen next. He wants to reveal our future to us so it builds our faith and trust in Him as we enter these end times.

He reveals your Path. He restores wisdom, love, light, energy, truth and spiritual connectedness with others. It is what "Idiosyncratic Core and Path" is all about!

Your **True Self** and **Life Purpose** were genetically installed in you before birth. God wants you to allow this process to reveal your True self, restore your Core and Guide you on the Right Path—this will create a life of balance and peace for you and the people you touch every day. When we try to control the outcomes of our Family, Friends, Work or Philanthropy we create conflict. When we go about it with a counter-intuitive mindset to let go and allow God to control the outcomes and timing in our lives and by putting in guiderails to keep us on Path—we live a balanced, peaceful, healthy, purpose-driven fulfilled life.

It is absolute necessary to know that God will never have you go through this journey alone. If you trust Him, He will bring people into your life's path as a rudder to help guide you through this turbulent storm you are experiencing and the restoration of your Core and Path. God is: just, loving, smooth, focused, gentle and strong.

This book should expose the evil in religious moral conformity as a way of finding peace or fulfillment and gives you a *self-discovery process* for your faith, a practice *for letting go and letting God* save you from yourself. This process is very powerful and simple.

Yet because most of it is counter-intuitive, it requires help to get there. This could be just the fuel your faith needs so you don't fall right back into your old life again.

Finding your predestine Chosen Path will change your life for the good and will resonate within your heart, but at the same time be counter-intuitive to your mind.

You need to be able to hold these seemingly diametrically opposed ideas in your mind at the same time. It is important to understand and respect these two powers – your sinful human evil desires and God's redeeming power that can save you from yourself. Your Ego-self does not want you to give up control of your life and become vulnerable to faith.

> *"The mark of a true genius is the ability to hold two seemingly contradictory ideas in mind at once."*
>
> – Albert Einstein

The healthiest minds are idiosyncratic and unpredictable as they follow the Path of self-discovery. This book will show you how to discover your Idiosyncratic "Core & Path" and walk with God in truth, while living in today's unstable world.

You cannot truly understand or appreciate anything until you experience it yourself! That's why this book is only for you who have "hit the wall" or "have been taken to the edge" or "come to the end of your rope" in order to break through your analytical Mind getting to your True Core deep in your heart.

CHAPTER ONE

Concentric Life Rings

Family and Friends Life Ring

In your relationships with family and friends, the first ring closest to your Core, we all need to let go of the outcomes that you feel are right for them. It's ok to start raising a child by constantly protecting them and their daily outcomes. But as they grow through childhood you have to let them use the gift of choice to make mistakes. With most humans success breeds repetition! That's why from thousands of paradigms in our minds, we are so blinded by our own success paradigms we can't see the "forest through the trees" let alone the Path to take.

But failure breeds change. It allows us to question our mindsets and trust someone other than ourselves. Someday each one of your friends and family members will come to the end of their own ropes and if they trust in God's mercy, they will break through their minds wall to their Core. In reality the edge is exactly where everyone needs to go. It is not about pushing people to the edge, but allowing them to go to the edge driven by their own desires. You can trust that God will be there on the other side to catch you and start the transformation process if you truly "let go."

Our responsibility is to be by their side — to be *kind* to them — not judgmental. The Bible says, only God's kindness brings people to repentance, not the law. The law takes you to the wall of despair. Healthy relationships with family and friends are always reciprocal—not a one-way street. So be careful helping family or friends in a one-way relationship. If either of you feel it is one-way, someone will end up feeling used or controlled, then they will probably resent you later. You need to slowly change from being a parent to fostering an adult relationship with your children. If you don't, you hold them in that parent-child relationship when they should become an adult.

The willingness to change your personal habits to meet the emotional needs of your friends and family member, especially your life partner, will be very effective. Are you finding that all the rings in your life are in conflict with each other? Does it seem like you have so many responsibilities that you don't have time for yourself?

This book could be your lifeline as God starts to transition your Core. The light of truth, if you let it into your dark center, will transform your Core and will give you a light to guide you on your new Path.

It is critical that you understand that your Path is not anyone else's Path. Each person's path is idiosyncratic. You shouldn't direct them or try and control their outcomes. You can only help them see God's work in your life. You can only offer them guide rails, humble support and wisdom. It's important that we do not take on the issues that they need to face themselves.

One thing my daughter has learned from clinical psychology. Is that you have to go to the level where people are protecting their Core, but you can't take on their issues. You may *feel* better about yourself, but that does not help the other person.

They won't hit their own wall of transformation. You are actually keeping them from breaking through their mind's wall to the light of restoration.

You should focus on your Core rather than fixing someone else's. Your actions speak louder than you words. So let God do the teaching. You will then be an example of enviable happiness for those you love. It is easy to forgive the ones you love, if you're not trying to correct them or control them. You can only truly love somebody when you care about him or her and respect them and their "Idiosyncratic" Path. You can't pretend. Only with Agape' (unconditional) love from God — can you truly forgive them.

Be *selective* with the people you let into your life because they affect your Core and Path development more than you think. As your mother would say, be careful about who you hang around with. Do your friends and family know what is truly important to you? If you don't know what is truly important to you, others won't respect your Core or Path.

Work Life Ring

Learning what to let go of at work is critical. Even though you are paid to control certain outcomes, you need to try not to control all the outcomes, at every level. It is critical to clearly define what you should control and what you should just influence or guide. Everyone at different levels in any organization feels responsible to control all the outcomes for the organization. No one can control all the detail and will hinder development of the organization if they do. That's true if you are on the management team or even one of the owners. There are too many other variables outside of the business structure that you cannot control. The future you try to strategically plan will not turn out the way you planed it anyway. Most people think that you or somebody in the organization needs to control your employees, your boss, customers, other departments, vendors, etc.

Even the strategic planning process used in business has you planning what you think you can control, only to find out later your customers, employees and economic conditions can change the final results no matter what you try and control. What typically happens in strategic planning is that you don't challenge the critical assumptions up front that the plan is based on. You end up building the plan with all the key milestones in place and the resources to implement the plan with absolute perfection. You end up building the plan as if you control all of the internal and external outcomes, only to find yourself surrounded with issues during the plan year that definitely affect the results.

There's a newer planning process that has helped many organizations build a better strategic plan. It's called the dialectic approach to planning. In this process you define five key strategies based on the key issues that need to be addressed. You discover your key issues by making a condensed list of your Strength, Weakness, Opportunities and Threats that you find out from both internal and external feedback. The best source is from the major stakeholders affected by the plan. After you have boiled down the extracted information that you feel will address the critical issues that next year, articulate five major strategies addressing the supporting data that you believe are facts.

Next, through a dialectical process of challenging what are truly supportable facts and what are assumptions, you expose and clarify the opposing thoughts to the assumptions. From those opposing assumptions you define five new counter strategies.

From those ten strategies you need to narrow it down to the five best major strategies to build your plan from. Many times at the end of this process, your leaders will choose their counter strategies.

See "Dialectical Approach to Planning" diagram at back of book in Appendix.

The counter strategies are the exact opposite of what they were going to build their plan on; building a more solid realistic plan that would define objectives, barriers, action plans, resources, milestones, timelines, and then a believable contingency plan.

The problem with this whole process is that you actually start to believe you can control the outcomes of customers, vendors, employees, and the external economic effects to your well executed plan. The problem is there are more issues out of your control than in your control.

Some people try and use a similar process when they try and go to sleep. They can't stop trying to think through every possible situation in minute detail, believing that their mind can protect them from situations turning out badly for themselves and their loved ones. Believing that if they can do the right things they can control the outcomes they desire. The problem is: it's not the truth. You might be able to control some of the outcomes, but the damage you cause along the way isn't healthy for yourself or others that you affect.

You can influence more than you can control.

In the same way people need to start addressing their rings and focus on their Core and Path, you need to do exactly the same with your business or career. Most companies as they grow larger through acquisition develop Cores that are misaligned and lose their clearly defined and articulated Path. Their Cores and Paths get fragmented. They believe, just like in your personal life, if they can control the outcomes, their Core will become healthy. They believe that if they can try and control all the outcomes, they are better leaders. This is not true for any of your life rings. It is all about addressing the Core of your business or your career and setting guiderails in place to keep you on your narrow Path.

Most people don't want to deal with that, because you might, for example, have to face the fact that some of your strong leaders at the top, or some of your big customers/givers that you are trying to please, need to be pruned away so you can get alignment. This will dramatically affect the organization, but it needs to be done to get to a healthy Core.

Any organization that has gone through a growth stage or been stagnant for a long period of time needs to address this. You should not be trying to please every customer or member. You should work to get alignment of the Leadership Core and Path with articulated focus, getting all the stakeholders (investors, employees, members, customers, vendors, and even other allied leaders in your venue) knowing how to invest their precious resources with you for a reciprocal benefit. It's a multiplying effect. One plus one can turn out to equal three!

The more people pushing in the same direction, the more powerful you become. It's about the influence you can have in your workplace when you have a focused Path and influencing from a strong Core. If it becomes apparent that where you are working is not aligned with your personal Core and Path, God will open a door for you in another direction. You don't have to try and make it happen. Just ask and then trust Him. Don't try and take control of the outcome.

The more power you try and give away or push down into the organization, the more power and responsibility will be given to you in your work life ring. It allows authority to go down into the organization instead of being controlled from the top. Most people believe that power or authority is appointed to someone at work—not earned. That's why tribal structure is hard to follow with a typical corporate structure. You should not lead with the concept of "Here are the rules. Here is the way we have to go."

It's more about the organization being aligned, than doing the right things from a perfect plan. It's more about putting the right structure together so the best plan of action can be implemented. Often the structure is that there is just one leader at the Core. Even God has three entities to sustain a balanced Core. Every person at the top should be in alignment with the Core and Path to allow stakeholders to invest with confidence. Allowing the Core management of an organization to stay misaligned with one another repels good leaders, employees, vendors, customers and investors.

Some of the same principles apply with big customers. Most people think that you should prepare in detail for what you think will make them happy by showing them the Path before you have aligned with their Core. They believe the person who thinks that the most complete presentation given to the customer will win the deal. Instead, if you make sure the they know you have spent the time to understand them and their issues they will trust you to lead the relationship.

They will allow you to lead them as a partner in a reciprocal deal – meaning good for both parties. Nobody wants to be sold, but everybody wants help developing his or her Path. Core alignment for an organization with a focused comprehensive Path will help all stakeholders align with you. Remember they can't align their resources unless they understand where they fit within your structure.

When it comes to leadership, especially the higher you go in an organization, your communication needs to be calmer and softer but direct. Your voice carries so much weight that even when you give suggestions they might see it as a command. People then may start using your name to get things done for themselves. Everyone you work with is looking for a leader. No one is looking to be controlled, so you have to be careful. The ultimate authority and leader is God. People even get mad at Him for not controlling things that affect their lives.

Laziness and pride cause the most damage in your work life. You can also see these as fear and entitlement. People can become paralyzed in fear: fear of making mistakes, losing their job, being late with a project or failure in business objective outcomes. Fear slows down productivity. Insecurity in people normally results in defensiveness or can be perceived as laziness or even pride.

Instead of keeping their nose to the grindstone and pushing the rock, they have their heads up looking around, off task and trying to manage the political landscape in which they find themselves. They will be working very hard to stay off the radar screen of management! All of these things lead to poor productivity and results.

Entitlement is there too. The people who find themselves acting entitled might say things like, "Why should I be the only one working hard? Other people get more recognition or money than I do and they aren't working as hard?" As entitlement grows people slow down their productivity, feeling they have earned the right to coast. Perhaps you give people awards for doing work that others in your organization, don't feel deserves it and as a consequence everyone can actually become more lazy and or prideful in your culture.

The most productive mindset for you and the organization is precisely in the middle between fear and entitlement, or between pain and pleasure. Too much fear and you will freeze like a deer in headlights; as you don't want more emotional pain. On the other hand with too much pleasure or feeling of entitlement, you become lazy and content.

All sins are reparable except believing one is without sin. If you believe you have done nothing wrong, you are in a precarious place. By exposing what you don't know or have done wrong, it allows others to help you. If you hide your weaknesses or failures from your vendors, employees, customers or stakeholders you will burden yourself with unnecessary worry that if they find out, they will stop supporting you and leave.

For example, if you hide the fact that your customer won't get his order on time, and they find out too late to adjust expectation on their end, they will resent you for the trouble you caused them. Ninety-nine percent of stakeholders will work with you around your problem if are simply honest and humble with the truth. You are just working against yourself by hiding the truth. When you are willing to accept that you need help, then others can help you. God cannot even help you if you don't humble yourself and ask Him to take control of your outcomes.

If a person defends their Ego-self then no one can help them.

That's why psychologists say the only people they can't help, are the people that think they don't need help. The mind is our biggest enemy. It will tell you that you are doing the right things and deserving of the results we want for ourselves.

There is not one sin that is worse than another because all sins isolate us from God and others. It is important to come to terms with and expose our inner conflicts with others. Conflicts need to be exposed so they can be resolved. If your Core is aligned you can work through your issues.

I believe that conflict is the foundation of a healthy relationship when it gets resolved, because exposing them makes you challenge the assumed facts in our minds, therefore it allows for a solid foundation to build a strategic plan.

Choosing when to expose a new strategic path to people affected by the change is critical. Most leaders feel they need to figure it out completely first before they share it with those affected. They typically get them involved too late in the process. The more you hide the development work of your organization, the more of a problem you have during implementation.

The Key Philosophy for Relationship Development

If people do not know in their heart & mind that you have taken the time to understand them and their current pressures and where they are heading then you cannot influence them to reach a solution. Even if the solution helps them out of a problem that you can clearly recognize. We foster the growth of our relationships by challenging our assumptions and understanding expectations, while being aware of perceptions. Facts alone are not enough to act upon. They must be challenged and confirmed, but perceptions must be acted on as soon as possible. That's right – as soon as possible.

Philanthropy Life Ring

This ring is about giving back where you get nothing in return. The other rings—your friends, your family and your work life, as you invest your time you expect to get something in return. This ring, however, is about being willing to give to causes that you feel directed by your heart and expecting nothing back in return. It's about just letting it go with your precious resources of money and even more importantly your valuable time. It is caring more about others in need than your own desires. It's about giving to the community around you or this big world filled with need.

Philanthropy is where your heart is pointing and should be confirmed by others who care about you—not your mind. God's kingdom work is where your True Self is being called. You feel in your heart that it is what you should be doing with your time. It's giving of your time or your financial resources. Sometimes it's only your time that's needed. I believe you should focus your giving to where you can get engaged and not just giving financially without giving yourself personally.

In most cases contributing your time in supporting a non-profit organization so others can feel comfortable and motivated to give, has more lasting value and can be more powerful than just giving financially. The amazing thing about this work is that the right doors will open if you are on the right Path. If you are not on the right Path the doors won't open at the right time, making you will feel like you have to adjust your expectations. God's timing with these things is perfect. If you try and control the outcomes of God's kingdom work, the timing will not pan out well.

Attempting to do what you think is right for God and trying to control when you think it should happen, will normally cause conflict for others involved. It is better to be selective and patient with this ring. If not, you will be consumed with activity trying to please God while at the same time thinking it is good for your spiritual development. Your mind will try to make your Core feel right about your efforts. You will be so mentally consumed in the timing that you won't be able to see the right doors opening for your chosen Path. This goes back to trying to *do* the right things to be the right person. God wants you to let go and let Him restore you to *be* the right person at the Core so you start to *do* the right things in your life rings. You have to feel it in your heart before you start acting the right way.

This outer ring can be in conflict with the other rings very quickly, if it is not aligned with God's plan for your life and your life purpose. All three life rings need to stay in balance.

If your philanthropy becomes too important or too time consuming that it strips away your time and energy for your friends and family, it is not healthy. Either is allowing work to become overly time-consuming. It's only when these rings align because your Core is open to your True Self and your Life Purpose is in harmony across all three rings that you are able to move forward without conflict in timing or with other people in your life.

This critical outer ring of God's work, the giving back ring, is the most fulfilling to your Core if aligned with God's will. With the friends and family ring you get something back short term and long-term in your life. The most interesting thing about this outer ring is that you feel something in your heart – a sense of peace – without needing anything back for balance in your mind such as not needing friendship, not needing money and not needing *anything* in return.

It wasn't until I went to Africa where I met people with whom I could expect nothing back from, but it was there I found the most powerful return blessing of all—the payback of Agape' love— unconditional love and the seed of faith that changed my life forever. The beautiful thing about this ring is that you don't have to make this ring happen to serve God. God will open up the doors and bring His work to you, making it easy for you to get involved without conflicts within your first two life rings.

This is the biggest part—the largest ring. It will become the most powerful ring. God will align your rings for you. This outer ring is where God opens doors where you give your most precious resource—yourself. This is foundational to give your resources unconditionally, the way God wants you to give. This has the strongest positive effect on your Core.

If we are His children and give ourselves unconditionally from our Core; the real transformation will happen. If we are fortunate to become more like God when we are alive, we get to live a life that is happier— more connected and peacefully balanced. You will be so thankful that you have this Father that cares and is always there for you.

You just can't take the present sinful self and shift so quickly to be Godlike. Most Christians tend to forget Jesus is God. It is hard to get our minds around who God really is. It shows too much light against our Core. So we ask "What Would Jesus Do?" Instead, the saying should go, "How would I be if I was like Christ?" God doesn't want us to do Jesus things, he wants us to be like Jesus.

Again, it's counter-intuitive to the way we were taught, that doing things make you right or wrong, but thinking things doesn't. Jesus said: "If you think it in your heart, you have committed it in Heaven." The mind is powerful and accountable to God.

Most Christians believe Sin is something we avoid but God created Sin to help us to let go of trying to control our own lives. Our Ego-self wants to work out our own salvation. The Bible talks about how our works toward pleasing God is being like "filthy rags." The message here is that we can't transform our own Cores; even with help from other humans. That's why this is niot a self-help book. We can't become like God of our own efforts and desires. All we can do is let go and trust God. The more you can learn to let go, the faster you get to your true Core transformation. That's why when we finally die and truly let go of our life, we can be fully transformed to be like Christ, becoming part of God.

Just as the author of the song "Amazing Grace" and Paul the Apostle saw themselves as worse sinners the older they became. Where you get into problems is when you think that you are becoming more like God by believing you are meeting His expectations. The only thing that stops the Spirit of God growing in your Core is yourself. There's this constant battle of you being the God of your life or letting God take control. The good thing about Heaven is that we won't be in charge of our own life any longer. The only thing that takes you to your idiosyncratic wall is your own natural Sin.

Conclusion of Life Rings

All three of these rings are strongly inter-related but need a clear separation from each other and be bridged by your life purpose. If your life purpose is succinctly written from your True Self and can be clearly articulated, you will be the exact same person in each of those rings. Most people think they have to adapt their behavior to each of these rings, but this causes conflict at your Core and with others around you.

See Life Rings diagram at the end of book in Appendix.

Discovering Your Core

What is your Core and how does it relate to the Rings

Right at the center of your three concentric life rings is your Core. At first look inside your Core you see what the mind can see: your Ego-self. What is not evident to your mind is that your True Self is hidden. The bible and our culture have many terms for this Core: heart, bowels, mind, spiritual center, soul, inner being, inner eye and many others.

Most people want to feel worthy in their mind, thinking that if they do the right things in the rings of their lives their Ego-self will find peace and happiness in your Core. But you won't find peace or happiness in controlling the outcomes of your life rings. Going on a missionary trip or a spiritual trip to Tibet won't insure you finding your True Self. Going to church twice a week won't guarantee you find your True Self either. Only your creator can provide the spiritual light of truth to reveal your True Self at the Core.

Your mind's Ego-self blocks your True Self from being exposed, because your ego does not want to lose the control it has worked so hard to get over the years. The key to unlocking your True Self is to break through your mind's wall to your Core. The problem for our analytical minds is that only the Spirit of God has the power to help us break through to the other side of self.

God is spiritual light. This light will transform your Core if you allow it. That is where I like to use the phrase: "you must die to yourself" to start this marvelous transformation. When you allow this light powered by Grace into your dark neglected childlike part of you, your mind starts to discover your True Self hidden deep within your Core.

I can only assume that you are reading this book because the Spirit of God Himself has put this in your hands and you're finding yourself at a point in life where you feel like you have hit a wall or come to the edge with no way to turn back. You might feel like you're drifting out in a vast ocean with no land in sight or that you're being controlled by God's powerful river of intervention and you have no energy to fight the current. You feel like your life is coming to an end the way you knew it. No matter how you got to this point in your life, thank God this is His way of reconciling His creation. Because He created time that allows change and He gave us choice, God had to give us the Law, which exposed sin that in turn separated the creation from the Creator. Until our naturally sinful selves take us to the place of self-destruction, our Ego-self won't let go of protecting our Core. This is God's perfect love based plan to rescue and restore what He had created with a free will to love and trust for Him.

Transformation of the Core

Life's best pathways to the marvelous transformations almost always come as a surprise. The untransformed can't invent their own path to transformation. It is rather the Creator who has the power to light the path and the grace to mercifully light the way. Through His mercy, He is willing to forgive us and direct us by His love and kindness to follow the Path He has embedded in us. Our job is not to figure out our future Path. Our job is to just walk in that light—to live our lives in that light every day. God will reveal our Path to us at the right time to build trust in Him, our caring Father. That's why when we say Jesus is the Light of the World it is a divine light of truth, not an earthly phosphorus light. It is not a search light through earthly advisors and emotionally motivating "self-helpers." It is not the seemingly light of truth that some self-help gurus profess will show you the way.

There are the worldly influences that are keeping us from the edge and God's wonderful restoration process of our Core. Your mind believes it is protecting your Core from hitting the wall. Self-help processes are a veil that blinds you from the truth that only God can restore your Core. For example, alcoholics need to accept who they are before they can start the recovery process. Sin makes you blind from seeing the truth about yourself. That's why if you have not hit the wall of truth about yourself, you cannot see that you are helpless on your own.

The reason so many people engage in self-help programs is because they don't want to let go of the end of the rope—they don't want to die to their Ego-self. That is too much risk for the mind, because it takes child like faith to let go and trust that God will be there on the other side to catch you. If I didn't have a stroke to soften my heart, if I had not gone to Africa to have the seed of compassion planted in my heart, and my wife did not reject me through divorce then I would have been so in control of my Core, that I would not have let go. However, I thank God for He used the right things to help bring me to the wall to break through to His trustworthy hands.

Deep in your core you have your True Self and its link to the creator—you are "pre-wired" with this True Self that can let go and trust God. You are also programmed through DNA as a descendent of Adam with a self-protecting "Ego-self." It is not one or another. You need to understand – these two co-exist. God will give you the strength for your True Self to start eclipsing your Ego-self.

You cannot fully eclipse your Ego-self in this lifetime, but if you stay humble and control the only thing that you truly have power over — your Ego-self—you can find peace and happiness and joy here on earth. The word "Blessed" in the bible directly translated from the original text means to be enviably happy!

The Holy Spirit has inserted the Arc of the Covenant for a permanent connection with our True Self in all those that are transformed at the Core, so we can hear His voice in our hearts, if we listen and not do all the talking when we pray.

The Other Side of Self

If you look at your Core as having two pieces—your Ego-self and Your True Self—you will see these are dialectically opposed or in conflict with one another.

As God's light of truth enlightens your understanding about this fact, you start to see this pattern in all of His creation. Once you can see these two parts inside of you, it starts to expose the self-centered ego that is keeping you from humbling yourself to God's grace. It's exactly what's happening to this whole planet. It answers the question, "How can God be a God of Love and still allow all these bad things to happen?" He set it up this way from the beginning of time ... to give us the power of Choice. The creation of TIME is the critical ingredient! You need TIME to use choice. TIME is never stagnant. It erodes or heals. TIME exposes Truth.

We want to believe that all of this is true, but when our Ego-self is fully engaged in this temporal world, we don't feel the conflict. Fortunately God created the Law that gave sin power in our minds. This drives us to the edge or "The Wall." Christ and the Holy Spirit expose this conflict in our Core and He gives us a way to save us from our Ego-self.

There has to be this conflict or there will be no resolution of reconciliation. Without the conflict between these two dialectic parts of our Core, there is no finding the truth we all seek. Without time there is no need for choice, for faith, for trust and forgiveness. When time has ended nothing will change again. It will just...be forever. Time creates this patterned dynamic for the creation to be rescued by the creator. This is the only path out of this Core conflict.

The way our minds work is to not want that conflict. Conflict is the foundation of a transparent relationship with God. It's facing that we actually have human evil at our Core. It's like the 12 steps of AA, accepting the fact that you are an alcoholic and that you need God's help. It's accepting the fact that your Ego-self has to die. Just like Christ had to die on the cross to take on the consequences for our sins. The results of all sin, is death. The key to the door to let God's light of truth into your Core is to submit yourself completely to God's restoration process.

Jesus was born without the genetic sins of the father. But God incarnate was placed in Time. He had BOTH sides so God could experience the conflict, but not yield to it. In His case He was God and His divine spirit controlled His Ego-self.

He was the only perfect sacrifice. He was the only one that didn't have sin, so He could take on the sin of the world and at that time. Christ said at that moment in Time, "Lord, why are you forsaking me?" At that point He took on our sins and died.

> *That is why the LORD says, "Turn to me now, while there is time. Give me your hearts. Come with fasting, weeping, and mourning. Don't tear your clothing in your grief, but tear your hearts instead." Return to the LORD your God, for He is merciful and compassionate, slow to get angry and filled with unfailing love. He is eager to relent and not punish.*
>
> Joel 2:12-13

It is the foundation of the Jewish religion to be saved. God deliberately chose the Jews and Israel to receive the Mosaic Law, allowing their strong Ego-self to try and meet the Law. Over time they replaced their Faith of Abraham with the Mosaic Law, giving them the power in their minds to condemn others and feel justified in their minds. This self-developed ego created a veil, so they would be blinded from the truth. He put a "stumbling stone" in Israel's path so that they could not see the faith of Abraham in Christ. The faith of Abraham was given before the Law. Without this conflict and public rejection of Christ, salvation would not have come to the gentiles.

It was critical for Israel to reject the cornerstone of Faith and be cut off from the vine, so the gentile branch could be grafted into the vine of Adonai (God the Father). The Mosaic Law was introduced to condemn, not set them free from their ego selves. The Law did its perfect work in them as it does all of us: exposing sin and condemning all who are born into sin. No one has ever met the Law expect Jesus the Son of God (God Himself). No one was or is worthy to be in God's presence without the blood covering of God's loving sacrifice of Himself through Christ.

It is important to accept the fact that how you think things should turn out in your life, probably won't turn out that way. Most people believe the lie that if they do the right things and plan in detail how they want things to turn out for themselves and the ones they love, that it is possible to control the outcomes in the future. The downfall is that if they don't get the major outcomes they expected, they get depressed and normally look for a scapegoat to blame. Note that you don't have control over what will happen; you only have the choice and the power to control yourself. Accepting this is critical to letting go and looking at your Core with God's help. Truly forgiving people who have hurt you is also imperative to accepting yourself at the Core.

When you don't forgive others who have hurt you, you can't accept the truth. For example, children who are abused often think they did something wrong. You just bury it deeper. Additionally, it is not about blaming others. Instead it is about forgiving versus holding on to the pain. Until you forgive the people who have hurt you, you can't find your True Self.

One of the hardest things you need to do in this process is to ask for forgiveness from everyone you have hurt in your past. Not in an email or letter. God asked that of me. He put 35 people in my heart to call, tell them what was happening to me and ask them for forgiveness for my actions. Maybe it was one person for every year I was married. That would be God's style with numbers. Most of them responded by saying how thankful they were that I had called them and they did not realize that I knew how I had hurt them.

When you have come to a place where "your life has come to an end as you know it" you may have lost a child, a spouse, gotten a divorce, lost a job or a company or been diagnosed with a fatal disease. These are all situations that can take you to the wall and your mind feels helpless. This book was written for you as a lifeline to a divine process that God had planned for you to rescue your Core.

As you allow God's light of truth into your Core to begin His restoration process, you will start to identify your fears. Then you will start seeing yourself as others do. *The truth about your self will help set your True Self free.* By lowering your Ego-self's protective shield you begin listening to God's subtle voice and others who truly care about you. You will be more honest with yourself by facing and confessing your anger and pain, but most importantly your sin filled human Ego-self.

The door to your True Self will begin to open. Validating your future self is the key to revealing your Path. Faith is the foundation for alignment at your Core and hope for a healthy True Self blended with God's Spirit; are the cornerstone that's required to bring balance across your three life rings and to reveal your life purpose. At this point your human ego driven mind has to die or yield completely to allow your True Self the room to grow and if you allow God's process to do it predestine work. Your True Self will start to eclipse your Ego-self at your Core.

Your True Self is the muscle of faith that you must start to exercise daily. The spirit is unnatural. That's why you can actually get to the point in life where you can be so narcissistic that your True Self muscle is atrophied from so little attention. You can't even use it find your way.

Next, you need to embrace your True Self. You can't love others unconditionally until you love yourself unconditionally like God does, and be thankful for the merciful work God is doing to your Core. Unless you're so hardened from embracing your human evil Ego-self for years, becoming completely narcissistic and controlling of your life rings, you will realize that the True Self at your Core is the only part of you worth loving.

At this point you have a choice to reclaim your True Self and allow God to start His merciful transformation process on your Core. Some people might call this being born again, being saved, accepting Jesus, spiritual conversion, rescued from themselves, rescued from the world, rescued from Satan himself, receiving the Holy Spirit, letting Jesus into your heart or just giving up and letting go, dying to your Ego-self and letting the Creator rescue your soul.

> *Then Jesus went to work on his disciples. "Anyone who intends to come with me has to let me lead. You're not in the driver's seat; I am. Don't run from suffering; embrace it. Follow me and I'll show you how. Self-help is no help at all. Self-sacrifice is the way, my way, to finding yourself, your True Self. What kind of deal is it to get everything you want but lose yourself? What could you ever trade your soul for?*
>
> Matthew 16:24-26 (MSG)

Life Purpose

You were born with a life purpose. Even if you can't articulate it, you have had it embedded in you since conception. It's a gift from the creator that we are meant to bring to others for His glory. It is not a career or avocation, but it is the essence of who we are in everyday life, reaching our full potential as the crown of His creation. Your life purpose is part of God's master plan to have a critical effect on the people you touch. He has others in the world with similar life purpose outcomes, but not exactly like yours. Your Life Purpose is truly idiosyncratic to you. That's why when you are not "On Purpose" you will feel discontent and unfulfilled living your life.

When your True Self becomes balanced with your Ego-self at your Core, you will discover your idiosyncratic Life Purpose. The wonderful thing about discovering and articulating your Life Purpose Statement is that it will bring your concentric life rings into synergy and balance with each other. These rings become strongly interrelated, needing a clear separation from each other while being bridged by your Life Purpose.

Core Life Purpose is the key to your chosen Path. This is God's plan for your life and will never change during your lifetime. Only your True Self can reveal your Life's Purpose. No other person or persons can tell you your Life Purpose, not even your Ego-self. It's hard to analyze or rationalize it when it is revealed, because it is normally not in alignment with your current Ego-self. Most people won't see it as possible because it is outside your normal behavior and old mindset. Learning to respect the responsibility of this Life Purpose is critical to your happiness and the positive effect you will have on others. It will be your rudder for your True Path in this world of uncertainty, guiding you with purpose in each of your life rings.

My Personal Life Purpose Statement

"I am the patient coach who opens up the inner person and provides the spiritual and emotional support for those who have been chosen to lead."

Paul A Omdoll

Concentric Life Rings Summary Points

- When it comes to your family and close friends it's critical that you understand your Path is not anyone else's Path. Each person's path is idiosyncratic. You shouldn't try to direct them or control their outcomes; only offering guiderail support.

- The most productive mindset for you and the organization to be in at the workplace is precisely in the middle between fear and entitlement, or between pain and pleasure. Too much fear and you will freeze like a dear in headlights; as you don't want more emotional pain. On the other hand with too much pleasure or feeling of entitlement, you become lazy in your responsibilities.

- If people do not know in their heart & mind that you have taken the time to understand them and their current pressures and where they are heading, then you cannot influence them to reach a solution. Even if the solution helps them out of a problem that you can clearly recognize.

- We foster the growth of our relationships by challenging our assumptions and understanding expectations, while being aware of perceptions. Facts alone are not enough to act upon. They must be challenged and confirmed, but perceptions must be acted on as soon as possible. That's right – as soon as possible.

- Philanthropy should be the largest ring in your life. It will become the most powerful ring because God will align your rings for you to support this work. God will open doors where you give your most precious resource—yourself. It is foundational to give your financial resources unconditionally, the way God wants you to give. This will have the strongest positive effect on your Core.

- At first look inside your Core you see what the mind can see: your Ego-self. What is not evident at first is that your True Self is hidden. The bible and our culture have many terms for this Core: heart, bowels, mind, spiritual center, soul, inner being, inner eye and many others. Here and only here will you find your True Self!

- Your Life Purpose is truly idiosyncratic to you. That's why when you are not "On Purpose" you will feel discontent and unfulfilled living your life. When your True Self becomes balanced with your Ego-self at your Core, you will discover your idiosyncratic Life Purpose.

- As your life starts to come back together with activity in all the rings of your life, your friends and family relationships, work-life relationships and relationships in philanthropy or God's Kingdom work, the most important thing for you to do is to be honestly sensitive with your Core alignment relationship with God.

- Maintaining Core Alignment is easy when life is going good, but the real challenge is keeping your Core at a consistent spiritual healthy state by staying in humble contact with the Creator.

CHAPTER TWO

Two Sides of Self

"Breaking through your Mind to the other side of self"

Your Core self has two parts: Ego Self and True Self. The brain is connected with your Ego Self. We are all trying to understand how to have faith—how to think and do the right things to find peace in our lives. In reality we have to *shut* the brain off to tap into our faith to link with the truth.

Ego-self

This is about understanding what we truly are without God. Our ways are not His ways nor are we naturally one with God like some humans want to believe. We don't think like God thinks. We are born into a sinful state because of Adam's sin. We are born with a healthy strong Ego-self at our core for survival. Our Ego-self does not desire union with God. Our Ego-Selves desire power, pleasure, eternal life, peace, value in God's eyes, to be heard, respected, comforted and supported, always looking for the acceptance of our choices.

Your Ego-self is not all corrupted. It has a purpose. It does separate us from other parts of His creation. It drives us to survive and increase productively in this world. God wants us to hold a desire to be blessed in this life by Him, which is motivated by our ego. We are created in God's image with choice—and the one part that allows us to think we can be our own god—is our ego. This dichotomy is the perfect example that we are His crowns of creation. We are creatures that can choose to be our own god or submit willfully and completely to the Creator. This ego is so strong that it takes "Hitting the Wall" before it will let go and allow our True Self to submit to another power.

Human connectedness to information

Nothing fuels the Ego Self like the Internet. You are focused 24/7 on activities versus your True Self-discovery. It started with radio, then TV, and now the Internet and texting. Now you have video calling on your phone. Eventually we will probably have communication and entertainment linked directly in our brain. Then you will be able to feed your Ego Self directly without any interruptions.

Your Ego Self has been conditioned over the years by your mind to control situations to find peace at your Core. So the key is controlling the growth of your Ego-self. God says that He has created us to have the choice of blocking Him or simply accepting His Grace. God has a healthy secure ego. He says "I am the only true God, there can be no other gods before me; I can be the only

Lord in your life." God has created the power of law and sin to condemn our ego-driven selves. Because we are in His creation of time, we are either moving closer to being like God or evolving further away from the truth everyday. It is hard for any of us to accept the concept of allowing our Ego-self to die. It's unnatural and illogical.

That's why you who have "hit the wall" should feel fortunate that you have this chance to let go and look to God for help. The last thing your Core needs is a self-help book to back away from the edge. Your mind does not want to bring an end to your ego's control of your future. This keeps you from letting go at a Core level, although you will always have enough power to open the door to Christ and His redemptive power. Unless the Holy Spirit draws you, you will never die to your ego.

No mind ever wants to give up control. We are natural survivors. We were born into sin ... not faith. Dying to self is counter-intuitive to your mind's paradigms. You are just trying to save yourself when you work on your salvation or try to earn God's favor. All that does is develop a spiritual ego. For example, you practice speaking humbly. This still feeds your Ego-self, thinking you're controlling your image to others.

Put reality and your Ego-self into the mix with law and sin and you will find yourself moving closer to the edge. It took me to some enviable lifestyle levels in 50 years. I had a conversation recently with someone who had a close friend that was very successful. From the outside he looked like he was living the perfect life but he recently threw himself off of a tall skyscraper in New York City. Eventually your Ego-self will feel shallow and empty if left to grow too large. All of the stuff we desire to feed our ego is not really worth any value to our Core. One little crack in the armor and we can truly "flip out." Some people find themselves at the wall and refuse to let go of their selfish ego and take their own life and maybe others that get in their path of destruction. You do everything to control the outcomes in your life rings and when just one more thing falls apart, turning out different than the way we think it should, it pushes us.

But there is life after Ego death. It's about breaking through your "Mind Wall" revealing your True Self and your right Path. It's that *seed* of True Self that God put in you when you were born. As the Light of Truth shines on your Core, it exposes your Ego-self for what it is and it gives you the *power* to let go. So you're spiritual True Self starts to take over your Core Space. This is something we cannot do ourselves. Our Ego-self will not allow it to happen.

We can try with all the power and control our mind can offer, but it is still our Ego-self doing it. It is not God restoring it through His merciful process of restoration. But if you *choose* to let go, He will catch you. If you open the door, He will come in. He won't leave you abandoned in a sea of loneliness. He will be your best friend.

If you choose to fix yourself through a "self-help" process, negative issues will come out in other places in your life. So no matter how you try to control your Ego-self by trying to do the right things to influence the major outcomes in your life rings, you avoid the truth that you need to face your sinful self.

Evil has its place in God's perfect plan of redemption. With the law to give sin the power to condemn your Ego-self, it will take your life to the edge and with the help of the Holy Spirit you to can break through your mind's wall to your other side of self. With the apostle Paul, God helped him see Jewish law as a stumbling block for Israel to accept Jesus, the cornerstone of Abraham's faith. This rejection of Christ being the Messiah opened the door for the gentiles to have a personal relationship with the living true God.

The most interesting truth is that as we have been made in God's image with the power of choice, so that we can choose to accept our fallen Core and the need to be rescued by the Creator. The Law's purpose is to condemn us, not give us a path to acceptance by God. The key is to bring your broken Core to Him, choosing God's merciful love and kindness to save you from yourself.

This is what I mean by metaphorically dying to self to live!

This is "The Lie." This is the Big Illusion. Your Ego does not want you to see that your True Self and Ego Self co-exist. It does not want to lose control of self. We are talking about giving up control of self and surrendering your Core. If you lose control of self, will God be there? This is the big fear. But you will break through to a place of orderly peace at your Core. You truly will be re-born to your True Self.

The Ego Self who we all know and love has been protecting us all our lives. It protects us from doing the wrong things, so why would we stop trusting it now? The True Self is the part that comes alive through Faith. The True Self holds the vision of your future self and unlocks God's spiritual light embedded in your Core from birth. It is NOT part of your ego. That light, that spiritual seed in each of us, is the spark of the Creator Himself.

True Self

Your True Self is not controlled by thought or reason. That is why it is difficult to explain and manage. An example is a true Yoga enthusiast or spiritualist who promotes "Oneness" where you try to quiet your ego self and mind to allow your True Self to emerge. It's the same in most Eastern religions. The person needs to try and meditate by shutting down the mind and listening to their center or Core. The more you try and use your mind to control your Ego-self, the more it becomes threatened and sees this process of "letting go" as foolish and vulnerable. I don't believe you can accept God into your Core with your Ego-self. I believe you need to accept God through your child-like, trusting and vulnerable True self.

When looking at a situation with our eyes, we see things differently with our True Self verses with the Ego-self. The Ego-self takes a position of advantage for controlling the outcome. True Self can have the faith and trust that God is in control, waiting with eyes wide open to see what door opens next and for the Divine gentle push down your Path. The brain is hardwired to your Ego-self. We are trying to understand how to have faith—how to think the correct things. In reality we have to *shut* the brain off to tap into our faith. *This is counter-intuitive to our mind!*

Each of us has the seed that can be unlocked. To unlock that True Self, the key is the light of truth. The Ego-self does not have that key. Notice sometimes when people try to do the right things driven by their mind or their Ego—it doesn't work so well! Your ego won't *accept* God's grace for what it is; it wants to judge and reason everything.

Our True Self feels imprisoned by a path that is not fulfilling. Most who feel *stuck* in life, until they feel this imprisonment on their path, won't change.

The True Self knows the right path forward!

The Ego can't die totally while we are still living in this world, but it can start to yield its power by *letting go and trusting God.* God himself chose to die through his human part "the son of man," so that his spiritual True Self could be raised. He is asking us to do the same thing—to die to our Ego Self by letting go to live life more through our True Self. This is not about you doing anything but letting go and allowing His Spirit to restore your Core and Path.

For example, this is not about committing Core suicide. It takes Faith, Hope and Love to release your ego from the life long responsibility to protect you. Faith is counter-intuitive to the brain's justification of action. Power and discipline of the mind won't do the job.

If you've been put in situations that are leading you to a place of letting go of your life, this book can help.

Remember, I couldn't swim to the shore. Because of my stroke, going to Africa and being rejected by my wife. Collectively it *helped* me come to the end of my rope and "Hit the Wall." I didn't choose this Path. My ego self would *never* have let go of control of what I had built for so long. I prided myself on doing the smart things. I was doing well in this world but not content at the Core. But God helped me *hit the wall* and *shoved me into a raging river* for a month. It took this level of intensity for a month for me to "let go" and trust God completely with the outcomes. I finally believed I could get my life back on dry ground once the river widened and calmed down. People have said that I could have swum to shore at some point to get back to my old life in the world, but I did not believe it. So I decided to let go and trust Him with my life, now that I had messed it up.

The Arc of the Covenant was a channel used by God to communicate to His people. When Christ died and went to

Heaven to release the Holy Spirit, that Spirit became enabled to connect to our True Selves. Our True Selves are like the Arc of the Covenant because God cannot talk to your brain directly. He can't communicate through your ego. But He can communicate to a Core that has been linked to Christ through the power of the Holy Spirit. This is a choice you have to make with your True Self. It's like God has the software and the Holy Spirit is the wireless connection.

Christ is the router/modem and your True Self is the wireless remote communicator that can't be connected until you *"let go"* of yourself in faith and let God complete the connection. Your Ego-self will try and block that connection.

I believe today that when you physically die and if you have made that link to the Creator during your life, your True Self goes to Heaven and is fully transformed to be like Christ the God. Your Ego-self will die with your flesh. Your True Self will look backward and forward with compassion; helping you make better decisions. Your Ego-self was not created to do that.

In Greek or Hebrew there are about five words for sin yet we only have the one word: sin. In these languages, once you are saved, those sins you do every day aren't counted against you as death. That's why the Apostle Paul said, "Now you are connected with him, all things are accepted, but they are not expedient."

Do not fret. Your True Self will not try to control life's outcomes; it's opposite of your Ego Self. As your life purpose is revealed it will help you make choices and bridge your Life Rings without conflicts. Again, God's perfect timing and your relationship with Him will allow that. You will be able to make better choicesand eliminate conflict across your rings surrounding your Core.

True Self is the child within you that stops development when your Ego Self takes over. That's why Mark 10:15 says, "I tell you the truth. Anyone who does not receive the kingdom of God like a child will not enter it." Our True Self holds the child part of us that never grows old and cynical. Our True Self sees life differently than our relational Ego-self.

> *Truly I say to you, unless you repent (change, turn about) and become like little children [trusting, lowly, loving, forgiving], you can never enter the kingdom of heaven at all. Whoever will humble himself therefore and become like this little child [trusting, lowly, loving, forgiving] is greatest in the kingdom of heaven.*
>
> Matthew 18:3-4 AMP

When you are born into this world, you are born with an Ego-self that develops quickly protect us and help us get what we need to survive. A baby has an Ego driven survival mode within the first few seconds of life. The restoration of our Core with the Creator does not start until we allow God access into our True Selves, through the sacrificial shedding of sinless blood.

We tend to think that our True Selves are as old as our Ego Selves, but actually, our True Self matures unrelated to worldly time. It can mature in a spiritual realm to an adult level, but it never grows old. There is a battle in our Core between these two and that's why we need to let go and let God do His predestined work in us. When we are physically dead, our Ego-self dies with our corruptible body. Only our True Self survives human death. That is why we can only enter the Kingdom of God with our True Self. It is the humble, softer, thankful part of us that has been nurtured to grow strong and healthy by the Spirit of God Himself.

Everything is about a balance for survival. Even our ego with our narcissistic minds help us *do* things to protect us. The ego, however, doesn't want to be vulnerable but the True Self without control is willing to be vulnerable. Please firmly acknowledge that the Ego-self cannot truly let go no matter how much your mind tries to control it. It can pretend to do so through many Eastern religions and self help processes. But I believe only God's Holy Spirit draws you to be rescued from the edge. If you completely let go of your ego controlled life and break through the minds wall; you might feel like you have nothing to hang on to, or you are a drift with no land in sight. But soon you will be enveloped with faith and the feeling of peace that your mind will not comprehend. Your Ego has the power to block this process of faith with the minds ability to reason. That's why you can only come to the Father to be reconciled through child like faith.

The purpose of this chapter is to enlighten you to the truth that the Ego-self can masquerade as your True Self with no real change at your Core. All of your survival techniques for physical, emotional and spiritual needs are driven by your Ego-self. Jesus said you should trust the Father each day with our lives. We can't do this by trying to control our sinful selves working hard to be worthy and pleasing to God.

We must let go of our lives to trust God with our Core

Your Ego Self grows and develops throughout your whole life. Your True Self will not begin to eclipse your Ego Self until God's Spirit touches it and links with it to give it life. This is what Christians call "conversion" or "being born again." Only when we receive this connection from God do we have the power in us to truly start dying to our self-preservation.

There are a lot of people who have God in their minds and are driven to do the work of God by their ego driven selves. We have all seen preachers, pastors and spiritual teachers believing that they are the most connected to God and lack the humility, grace and compassion evident with a Core that has hit the wall of narcissistic behavior. They lead many people on a path that feeds their Ego Self at the Core masquerading as true peace from God. Why? Because your Ego searches high and low for truth and has no faith in future outcomes. It's why people are drawn to watch the news and see how frustrating it is for others in this world, so they feel some sense of peace in their lives. All of these things are self-driven by the Ego.

The key to finding your True Self is actually simple: Just accept that it must be exposed to the light of truth to be revealed. It's deeper than cognitive thought. It's also found when you stop talking with yourself in your mind. It is at the center of the Core of our being. Controlling our Life Rings only exposes the Ego-self. True Self will be the rudder in your new life, keeping you on your balanced enlightened Path. It knows what and when situations are not right for you in your life. Your True Self is not in conflict with God's will for your life. Your Ego-driven desires can and will override your True Self quite easily and brutally. Once you have a focused *"Life Purpose"* revealed by your True Self, you will feel the courage to live out your life's purpose. Your Ego-self tells you that you are not prepared, or you don't have enough information to risk the loss of control. It's too difficult or you will need it in the future ... just not now. You be will be too vulnerable!

Your True Self gives you certainty, hope and a peace that's beyond understanding. It confirms to your mind when you are on the right path and when you might take the wrong path. Say for example, you are between jobs and you finally get that great job offer you've been waiting for but your True Self tells you, surprisingly, not to accept that job. It allows you to stay on your path and hold course within the guiderails. You must have faith in God's perfect timing in your life. It will happen just when He wants it to happen, having the most positive effect with everyone affected by the outcome, including your self. Our choices tend to have trade offs. Having enough patience is the rough part. We have to learn to wait on God and not get ahead of Him. Our Ego has a hard time with this part of the process!

Finding a quiet place where you can listen to the voice of God; that small voice in our True Self, your Ego Self will try to talk over it in your mind. Your True Self is the child at your Core. It can mature slowly to an adult state with God's help, but it will never grow old. This is the part that never dies and will live forever in eternity.

Barriers to True Self

What are some of the barriers to developing your True Self and finding your chosen Path?

- *Choosing the outcomes that the Ego-self Desires*
- *Planning moves to get desired outcomes*
- *Trying to control major outcomes in your lives rings*
- *Trying to control the outcomes of those you love*
- *Not trusting God's guidance and letting life happen*
- *Ignoring your spiritual journey your whole life*

Most managers, leaders or parents try to control the outcomes of the people they feel responsible for, more than being concerned about the alignment of the core people or staying on Path. It is the same in your own life. Most people think that bad situations or closed doors are taking them off their path. It may be getting you back on the right path. That's what faith is about! It's counter-intuitive to your brain. As I read somewhere, "a bad year in your life is a good year for your soul."

"Who and Where" is your choice!

If you are in an environment that is calm and accepting of who you are, or with someone that loves you just the way you are, you don't feel the need to defend your insecure Ego-self for survival. This allows your Ego-self to back down because it is not needed to protect yourself, allowing your True Self which is the kind, caring, thoughtful, giving, forgiving part of your ***"Self"*** to come out and share your open and honest heartfelt feelings. This is how God's Grace works. If God will accept you just the way you are as a natural born sinner, you have a chance to stop defending your Ego-self and allow God to start the reclaiming process of growing your spiritually centered True-Self.

I have noticed that the Holy Spirit most days likes to connect with your True Self early morning before the sun comes up. I believe your mind and Ego-self are more likely to block the connection with logic and reason to counter-intuitive spiritual truths. Yielding to this connection each day allows you through a spiritual direct link God has created through His Holy Spirit to connect with your True Self engaging His predestined restoration process. The mind and Ego-self are the barriers to this live on-line connection with the Creator.

The best way I have found to make a solid connection is to not do most of the talking in my mind. Start by acknowledging who and what God is. The living God, Creator of all things, is *pure* love, light, power, and energy. He is the only one that knows the future because He is outside of time. You will know when you're connected when this feeling of a warm rushing sensation pours over you like a spiritual orgasm. It is truly a two-way direct connection with God the Father. You can sense the power of the creator, the love and peace of the risen Christ, and the power and presence of the Holy Spirit.

Your Ego Self does not desire a union with The Creator, but it does desire His power and support of our desires. Even if we desire to do God's work for Him! Your Ego Self is the part that prays for things that you think God should help you with. The True Self only wants God's will to take control of situations. Your Ego-self which is in conflict with your True Self, is conditioned by your mind to think that you need to control people and situations to find peace at your Core.

When your mind tries to understand the True Self that God starts to reveal; you will find that you are not the person your conditioned mind thinks you are.

This book is an instruction manual of God's process after you *"Hit the Wall"*

If you let go and trust God to take you through this process, He will!

Two Sides of Self Summary Points

- Your Core has two parts: Ego Self and True Self. The brain is connected with your Ego Self which is the logical adult, developed of paradigms from assumed facts. The heart or soul is connected to the True Self which holds the vulnerable inner child with faith to believe in the unknown.

- Our Ego-self does not desire union with God. Our Ego-Selves desire acceptance, power, pleasure, eternal life, value in God's eyes, to be heard, respect, peace, comfort, support and acceptance of our choices. It tries to control your mind, and tells you what you think you should *do*.

- God has created the power of law and sin to condemn our ego-driven selves. Because we are in His creation of time, we are either moving closer to being like God or evolving further away from the truth every day. It is hard for any of us to accept the concept of allowing our Ego-self to die. It's unnatural and illogical.

- The key to life's door to the other side of self is to metaphorically die to your Ego self. Your Ego does not want to accept that your True Self and Ego Self co-exist. It does not want to lose control of self. This is "The Lie." This is the Big Illusion. We are talking about giving up control of self and surrendering your Core. If you lose control of self, will

God be there? This is the big fear. But you take the step of faith; you will break through your minds wall to a place of orderly peace at your Core.

- Each of us has the seed that can be unlocked. To unlock that True Self, the key is the light of truth. We are trying to understand how to have faith—how to think the correct things. In reality we have to *shut* the brain off to tap into our faith. *This is counter-intuitive to our mind!*

- Your True Self, the other side of self, is not controlled by thought or reason. Wait with your eyes open for the Divine gentle push down your Path. Just *be*. Turn off your brains and tap in your inner faith and trust God. Don't tell yourself, "I will try to trust God" – simply know it in your heart and you will radiate your belief.

- Most managers, leaders and parents try to control the outcomes of the people they feel responsible for; more than being concerned about the alignment of the Core of the leaders or the family unit. It is the same in your own life. Most people think that bad situations or closed doors are taking them off their path. It may be getting you back on the right path. That's what faith is about! It's counter-intuitive to your brain to let go and have faith.

- The purpose of this chapter is to enlighten you to the truth that the Ego-self can masquerade as your True Self with no real change at your Core. All of your survival techniques for physical, emotional and spiritual needs are driven by your Ego-self. Jesus said you should trust the Father each day with our lives. We can't do this by trying to control our sinful selves working hard to be worthy and pleasing to God.

CHAPTER THREE

Core Transformation

Core transformation is not something you can do or perform yourself. That is why this is not a self help book telling you or teaching you how to fix your Core and Path. The Core transformation I am talking about comes when you are willing to let go of protecting your Core from His grace through faith alone. How can you tell His Grace is calling you? If you sense a major loss of control in your life or find yourself wanting to escape the pain your choices in life have put you in. You should realize that that desire of wanting God to intervene is not something your Ego-self could have generated. This process requires help from an outside power. If this is happening to you at this time, this book was prepared for you because of His love for you through me. If you are still holding on tight to your life's outcomes and have not "Hit the Wall" yet, this book will be hard for your mind to understand or accept.

What is God saying to you?

Is God saying to you to follow Him beyond what you can control, beyond where your own strengths and competences can take you, and beyond what is affirmed or risked by the crowd around you? If this is resonating in your heart and you let go and trust Him completely, you will experience God's Power, Wisdom, Grace and Unconditional Love; more than you could *ever* imagine the Almighty God paying you so much personal attention.

God is calling you to follow Him to a place of weakness where you risk the vulnerability of a child, so that you might know how strong the Father is and how much He loves you!

There are many Christians who want their hearts and minds transformed to be like Christ, but they can't seem to let go of their lives of selfishness and pride only trusting God's grace to allow the transformation to take place. The Bible says no man seeks God. Only the Holy Spirit can draw you to want to face God with your Core and True Self that has been asleep in you since your birth. That's why this book is not a self-help book. I'm encouraged knowing that our ego, our sinful desires, and our life choices will take us to the Wall. It is only when the Spirit helps you break through your own ego developed mind and let go, can this process of restoration take place.

No human mind wants to "let go" and die a metaphorical death!

This is why it normally takes a tragedy in someone's life to literally "*let go.*" Your ego does not want to lose control of your Core. It's like people on a Yo-Yo diet. They go up and down repeatedly throughout their entire lives. It is essentially a perpetual Tug-of-War inside their Core. A similar situation happens with most zealous religious people. They sin and repent, repeating this cycle over and over trying to do the right things to please God and their conscience or self-image. Even most Christian leaders try and teach their followers how to *do* the right things to please God, but they try with their minds to control their sinful lives and thoughts—all to no avail—because our righteousness through our own efforts is like filthy rags in God's perfect eye. This process of sin control actually keep us from the edge of letting go in faith, while all the time God is trying to bring you to the Wall—the Wall of breakthrough to the other side of self—your True Self.

Following a list of "do's and don'ts" usually result in either self-righteous pride, if you think you are achieving it; or secret shames if you feel like you constantly are falling short.

It tends to drag you through an endless cycle of shame and guilt: "I've sinned again and shamefully regret it" leaving you feeling like you owe God a debt and want to pay it back. So we think that we have to do something ourselves to earn God's favor back. Then we are motivated to do extra good things for awhile, this helps to alleviate some of the guilt and gets us away from the edge or wall but ultimately we go right back into the shame cycle.

What happens to most humans is that is we are stuck in this cycle long enough, we end up believing we are totally bad at the Core, saying to ourselves we are hopeless, "I am it" (I am the alcoholic, the addict, the loser, the problem). When this happens we ignore the truth of how God sees us as His lost child and the open door of grace seems locked because of believing that our evil is more powerful than God's grace. There is no grey area to stand in: we are committed to Him or our sinful selves. There is no other choice!

> *"There is no neutral ground in the universe: every square inch, every split second is claimed by God and counter claimed by Satan. We must choose one enslavement or the other; we have the choice and the will!"*
>
> – CS Lewis

If you read Romans a few times and understand what the Apostle Paul is trying to communicate to his own people, the Jews, you will see that God planned to have sin do its work in us so the Law could condemn us, not give us life through meeting the rules. Christ was teaching the laws of Abraham's faith rather than the Jewish laws of control; that's why the Jewish leaders wanted Him dead. The Jewish leaders of Israel did not want to give up the hierarchical control that the Mosaic Law and the laws that they added over the years to give them power and control over each other. If they would have *"let go"* and followed Jesus like Paul the Apostle, the Jewish hierarchical structure would have collapsed.

The catholic/apostolic structure that most Christian faiths are based on would have the same problem today of 'letting go."

An intellectual obedience to God's Law can serve as a wall for rebelling against God.

The apostle Paul points out that the Pharisees who try and uphold the Law with perfection still break the Law. God removed the vale from some of the Jews so they could see the truth, but the majority were given a stumbling stone so they would reject Christ as the Messiah. This was God's Divine plan to open the door of salvation through giving of Him self at that time to the rest of the Gentile world through the rejection of the Messiah. Most Jews are still looking for the Messiah today to lead them to a place of power in the world, but it is not about the power on this Earth. It is about the power of God's Spiritual Kingdom and our idiosyncratic personal relationship with Him through a humble faith based transformation.

We must die this *metaphorical death* at our Core for the seeds of faith that have been planted through the miracle of birth and God's purification process of binding with our spiritual Core to start His reconciliation process. This transformation process of dying a metaphorical death is just like how a forest is reborn after a forest fire.

There are certain pinecones on each tree that are designed to go through the fire and open up after the death of the tree to restart the forest. Many pine trees are dependent on forest fires for ecological survival. Many species develop thick bark at an early stage in their life cycle. This turns out to be a benefit during a forest fire, for these pine trees will survive the fire, while other competing trees, especially hardwoods, will not. These pine trees have cones that are defined by botanists as being serotinous. They are naturally sealed shut by resin, but during a forest fire the heat will melt the resin and release the seeds from these combustible pinecones. None of these species produce a crop of cones that is completely serotinous.

This is just like God's plan of reconciliation. Many are called but few are chosen to have the seeds of Faith after they *"hit the wall."* Their lives have gone through the cleansing fire directed by the Holy Spirit, only for God to finish the work that He started, bringing new life full of blessings.

You can't save anyone. You can't spiritually rescue anybody. But you can help! He can use you to help rescue others. It's not uncommon that He will use you to rescue someone you don't know well or not at all. Many people try to rescue their families or loved ones unsuccessfully. God can't rescue anyone that doesn't accept that they need rescuing. The Ego Self does NOT want to go to lose control and go to the edge. We think we are pleasing God by staying away from the edge of faith. We have to accept that we have a strong human evil ego to let go. I realize we don't want to think of ourselves as evil or bad at the Core, but through God's Grace we can *"let go"* so God can do His predestined work in us. This process is hard for our minds to accept because He created us in His image. We have the power of choice and this alone can keep you from God's wonderful reconciliation plan of spiritual Core transformation.

If your True Self is rescued and restored by God, you can begin to see your Path blessed by Him with the light of truth as your personal guide.

Your spiritual growth during your personal transformation will speak volumes about your heart for God and how your gifts and energy can impact the Kingdom of God. Those closest to you will need time to accept and respect those Core changes. The baggage of the past will still hang around the corners of their perceptions, so you'll need patience with their "learning curve."

> *"If you follow the protocol that God is unfolding in your life, there will be sustaining transformations that some will not see, because they were too close to the "your old Self." And they will probably need to test the credibility of your new commitments and grow to respect and give thanks as the past fades and your new True Self shines to glorify God."*
>
> – Richard Cobb

12 Steps of Transformation (taken from Alcoholics Anonymous)

1. We admit we are powerless over sin—that our lives had become unmanageable.
2. Believe that God can restore us to His will.
3. Make a decision to turn our will and our lives over to the care of God.
4. Make a searching and fearless moral inventory of ourselves.
5. Admit to God, to ourselves, and to another human being the exact nature of our wrongs.
6. We're entirely ready to have God remove all these defects of character.
7. Humbly asked Him to remove our shortcomings.
8. Make a list of people we had harmed, and become willing to make amends with them all.
9. Make direct amends to such people wherever possible, except when to do so would hurt them or others.
10. Continued to take personal inventory and when we are wrong promptly admit it.
11. Sought through prayer and meditation to improve our conscious contact with God, praying only for the knowledge of His Will for us, and the power to carry that out.
12. Having had a spiritual awakening as the result of these steps, we try to carry this message to others in sin, and to practice these principles in all our affairs.

In the same way that an alcoholic has to accept that they are powerless over alcohol and that their lives have become completely unmanageable, those who are willing to allow true transformation of our Core must accept this same fact that we are powerless over sin. As we start to examine our Core and peel back the protective shields of our Ego, getting to the truth of who we really are by taking a fearless moral inventory of ourselves, we enter into dangerous territory.

For our egotistical minds to accept that we embody such evil leaves us two critical choices—to either turn on ourselves which pushes us deeper into despair and depression or it allows us to open the door of faith and call out for a higher power to save us from ourselves.

It is also a critical step to allow God to bring to your heart and mind the people that you have hurt over the years while you have been living your Ego-centered life. The first step is not just making this list from your mind. It's not about a mental process. This is about asking and allowing God to reveal to you who He wants you to restore your relationships with. God loves to restore. We normally want to get this behind us quickly as possible to avoid the future pain, like quickly pulling off a Band-Aid. But it is God's perfect timing that you must wait for, as He might take a year to open someone's door to his or her heart for transformational healing. It is not just about you!

For me God actually had me call someone who knows the person I was to reach out to first. This was someone who knows that intended person really well. God had me call this person to "ask permission" to contact the intended person first before asking for forgiveness.

I have had some people say, "I would call this person now as it has been on their mind for a long time." Or they might say, "Now is not a good time, I would wait awhile." It's not just about getting release for your self. It's about the other person being exposed to God's hand of grace. It's also not about just wiping your hands clean of your past actions. This process opens the door to share what God is now doing in your life and how God is dealing with your sinful nature. It also helps you face the damage you have done and the consequences for your actions with a repentive heart.

In some cases people would respond to me, "I was not bothered at all by what you did, but it touches me because you took the time to come back and connect with me." It's about taking the unselfish time to care about someone else's life. God uses this care and love and kindness to touch them. Remember only God's kindness brings people to repentance, not His law. So when you go back and ask people for forgiveness, they should see this as this act as kindness. Your goal in this process should be to let these shadows of darkness face the light of God's healing love.

God's Restoration Healing Process

- *Redeem our past*
- *Heal wounds of those we've hurt*
- *Heal our life wounds*
- *Safeguard our families*
- *Purify our thought life*
- *Sanctify our ambitions*
- *Soften our hearts*
- *Comfort us through His wisdom*
- *Fill our minds with scripture*
- *Teach us to trust His Word*
- *Show us His love for us*
- *Reconcile our relationships (especially family)*
- *Then God's Spirit will lead us from being rescued to a rescuer*

Scripture is very clear that God loves to reconcile everything He creates. God planned to reconcile His creation before He started to create. What this statement means that if God planned to reconcile then He planned to create good and evil and the freedom of choice. Some people want to think that a good God wouldn't create the concept of evil. That Satan created himself. That would be the most evil deceptive lie. That would make Satan equal to God as a creator. God created everything. There is nothing that God did not create and plan. He is before all time and all things during, and after. He is the Alpha and the Omega. Nothing happens in time that God does not allow.

Once you understand that God is not limited by time, you can you trust Him to rescue you *in time.*

My Transformation

I have now experienced in my life the difference between accepting Jesus in my heart back when I was in my twenties as a desire to have eternal life and feel better about my sinful self, and now the experience of "hitting the wall" and triggering a spiritual awakening, which I have shared with you in the introduction of this book. I believe now that if I hadn't become as life hardened in my heart and not gone through the experience of my stroke, Africa and the divorce, I would not have let go completely to allow God to save me from myself.

When I was young I had always felt God was out there looking at me. Watching my every move, judging me from a distance with no parental care for my Core or Path. I guess I only knew God as this powerful disconnected creator. As I look back over my life and paths that I have taken, I can now clearly see that God was always there with a parental unconditional love, supporting me and protecting me even when I was far away from His unique Path for me. I knew He loved me, but I never really loved Him back. God says in scripture that if you love Him, you will obey Him. I was truly the prodigal son. I took the blessing that His love had showered me with and used them for worldly pleasure, feeding my Ego Self for over 30 years.

God loved me enough to stop allowing me to live an unfulfilled life without His direction and guidance. I desired God's blessings and offer of eternal life with Him later in Heaven, but chose to live my life the way I wanted. When I had made the choice to let God into my heart back then, I had held a few cards back to protect my Ego-self and a few worldly desires that I expected Him to remove from me later on.

As I share this concept with people, I find most people that are honest with themselves will admit the same thing. I now believe that until you "hit the wall" as a consequence of the predestined work of sin and the Law doing it's work of condemnation, you will keep trying harder to stay away from the edge of spiritual failure and take that leap of faith.

Most people that seek peace and comfort for their soul go through phases of spiritual failure for different reasons, only to find themselves over time feeling lost. I believe God knows how hard it is to die to yourself and truly trust Him to be Lord of your life. He is patient and full of grace. God is always right there to save us from ourselves, even when sin has caused us to hide from His unconditional healing love. This is not the end of my evil ways, but the start of a path of faith in a God that cares enough to enlighten my path with teaching through my idiosyncratic failures of seeking more knowledge than wisdom. Wisdom is seeking faith in a higher power and understanding we will always have the two dialectic parts of our Core until we shed our corruptible bodies. As the Apostle Paul said, "Who can save us from this evil person within us? Only a living God that has paid the price of sin as a perfect sacrifice?"

God continues to transform me from my sinful self. I believe this process will only stop when I die physically and become fully transformed in spirit to be like Him. Until then my life will be filled with failures & learning from choices emanating from my Ego-self, balanced by blessings growing out from my counter-intuitive True-Self made possible by faith and trust.

One Amazing Story

My cousin on my dad's side was a troubled soul for most of his life. He was a tall, well-built man that endured a rough life. He worked many hard jobs around this big country trying to find his place in life, from working on shrimp boats to capping oil wells. He had a drinking problem for the majority of his life and was seen by most of his friends and relatives as the troubled black sheep of the family. He had been in a few prisons during his middle years, but these were things that the family tried to sweep under the rug from embarrassment. He was considered as one of the bad guys in society, even joining a hard-core motorcycle gang in Milwaukee for a time. He lived the type of life that if he hadn't taken the life of at least one man during in his lifetime, I would be surprised.

At his funeral, a granola-type female pastor in sandals and a colorful robe from a local social church got up to give the liturgy, making the point that God is a loving God and everyone gets to go to heaven if you're a nice person, and even mentioned that from talking to his friends and family, she was sure my cousin was a nice person and went to heaven.

Then a special guest stood up and said she had to share what God told her to say. Her name was Kim and she had been sent by God to speak at my cousin's funeral. What she said touched everyone there that day. Afterwards I had asked her to send me the notes from her statement. She said she didn't really have notes, but she remembers what God told her to say almost word for word and she would type it up on a typewriter and mail it to me, because she didn't have a computer or email. So here is what I got in snail mail a week later. It was exactly the way I remembered it from my cousin's funeral.

God led me to speak here tonight. Gary was a good friend of mine and I loved him as my brother. Yes, Gary was a caregiver. He was always there for me, fixing things and always helping me with something. The first time I met Gary, he gave me a box of good tea, in different flavors. It was winter and I was always sick with a bad cold, so it was very nice. One night when I came home from work, I saw Gary in the hallway and told him I had to go grocery shopping, that I had nothing in the house for dinner. A couple of minutes later he was knocking on my door with a roast beef dinner for me. In the Bible, Jesus said, "Truly, Truly I tell you, if anyone among you gives to the least of these a cup of cold water; they have given it to Me. They shall not lose their reward.

Gary will have a lot of rewards in heaven." I wasn't sure where Gary went when he passed away. But, God assured me that when Gary was in the hospital, He visited him and saved Gary. I thought Gary would be coming back home, but I had a feeling Gary knew he wasn't coming back here. Gary wants to see all of you again. God loves Gary and He loves all of you. I'm going to give you an invitation from God to see Gary again and to have Eternal Life with our Father, Lord and Savior. If you want to know where you are going after this life – you can know for sure tonight. It is a matter of life and death. We don't know if we will be here tomorrow.

She then asked everyone to pray with her to let God save them and thanked God for forgiving our sins. Then she thanked everyone for letting her speak and sat down. We all sat there in shock! You couldn't ignore the contrast at the funeral between these two small women and our large cousin in the coffin; a social protestant granola type female minister and a simple uneducated common woman with a child-like faith that you couldn't emotionally hide from.

God's Spirit was there in full force that night. Only a hardened heart with a veil of self-righteousness over it could block the truth that filled the funeral home. After the funeral was over, she said to me that she knows God comes to you on your death bed and tries to reconcile you back to Him, because it happened to her years ago when she had basically died in the hospital. She told me that Jesus came to her that night and saved her soul, then she woke up and God started restoring her body that was giving up and shutting down.

About a month later Kim and I got together for lunch. We had a very spiritual and enlightening lunch together. First I believe the Spirit revealed to us a truth that could bring a sense of peace to many families that have lost a loved one. Christ comes to all at their deathbed and offers salvation. But, if they chose not to trust Him and keep holding on tighter to this life not accepting that they are at the end of life's rope, they won't let go to be rescued. God can't break their will, so He can't rescue those souls that reject His saving grace.

Because God is love and filled with grace! It is only logical that God would give the crown of His creation one last chance before they die. But if you don't want to let go of your Ego-self and accept His saving grace even on our deathbed, God won't force you to save your soul. Kim told me about her amazing story of God's intervention and how He saved her life here on earth and for eternity. She is such a sweet and humble person that it was easy to see that the story she was about to tell me, was going to be a recollection of the truth straight from her warm heart.

Kim O'Keefe's story of Transformation

It started back in Sept. of 1989 when she ate a salad from a fast food chain's salad bar only to find out later, the person preparing the food for the salad bar had "Hepatitis A" and she got infected along with a few other people.

Two weeks later she came down with flu like fever that wouldn't go away. Her urine started turning brown because "Hepatitis A" destroys the liver. She was in the hospital dying for a month and starving because she couldn't hold down food with her symptoms. Since Hepatitis A is a virus, it cannot be treated with any medication and her liver just kept slowly shutting down each day. Saving her seemed hopeless.

In November of 1989 one night in the hospital, when she accepted the fact that she was going to die, she cried out to God to save her. She thought there must be a father-like God in Heaven even though Kim had never gone to church her whole life. She told me that maybe she had gone to church as a child once on some religious holiday. She was born Catholic, so she only remembered seeing Jesus on a cross and thought He had died there, but didn't know about His resurrection.

While she was asking God how she could be saved and get to heaven, Jesus appeared outside her hospital room window. Then He appeared next to her bed wearing a purple robe. She said she could feel His overpowering love next to her. She asked Jesus to rescue her. He explained what she had to do to be saved by Him, so she spent an hour confessing her life sins to Him. He then told her that her sins were taken care of and she needed to change the way she was living. She told Him, I can't change on my own, but He told her he would help. *Then Jesus took her hand.*

He held her hand and said He could be with her forever if she let Him in her heart. So she did. Jesus spent the rest of the night holding her hand talking with her in her hospital room. She didn't sleep at all that night. She said she was scared that if she fell asleep, Jesus might not be there when she woke up. I had then asked her how she felt that night. She said she felt comfort, peace and security. She disclosed that they talked about all the past traumatic issues from her life and He promised her life would be different from now on. She remembers praying that no one would come into the room and interrupt this personal visit from God. She was surprised that no one came in that night, because they would normally come in and check something at least every couple of hours.

After that night, she was so happy in her heart, even though her body was getting worse. Her mother and the nurses said to her the next day that she seemed different. Slowly her symptoms started to change over time and to the doctor's amazement, she miraculously recovered. She told no one of this private meeting with Christ for one full year. This was just between her and God. Jesus would come to her every morning and taught her every day for the rest of that year. She was scared that if she told someone that He would not keep showing up each day. She was healed and is here today and healthy again.

So if God can forgive and save people on their deathbed, God can forgive and save you.

True Transformation is a Gift of Grace

True transformation has to be a gift, because if it wasn't it would have to be earned by good works and God's gift of Himself born by His love for His creation would have been unnecessary. This gift renews your mind, if you are willing to offer yourself as a living sacrifice. To receive this gift of transformation, we must make the choice to "die" to our old worldly mindset and opening the door to our Core to the Creator. Life's best pathways to the most marvelous transformations almost always come as a surprise! Remember, you can't invent your path to transformation because the Creator has the power to carve that path paired up with the grace to mercifully light the way He has planned for us.

Our job is to just walk in that light!

When we were controlled by our old nature, sinful desires were at work within us, and the law aroused these evil desires that produced a harvest of sinful deeds, resulting in death. But now we have been released from the law, for we died to it and are no longer captive to its power. Now we can serve God, not in the old way of obeying the letter of the law, but in the new way of living in the Spirit.

Romans 7:5-6

I have discovered this principle of life—that when I want to do what is right, I inevitably do what is wrong. I love God's law with all my heart. But there is another power within me that is at war with my mind. This power makes me a slave to the sin that is still within me. Oh, what a miserable person I am! Who will free me from this life that is dominated by sin and death? Thank God! The answer is in Jesus Christ our Lord. So you see how it is: in my mind I really want to obey God's law, but because of my sinful nature I am a slave to sin.

Romans 7:21-25

And since it is through God's kindness, then it is not by their good works. For in that case, God's grace would not be what it really is—free and undeserved.

Romans 11:6

Notice how God is both kind and severe. He is severe toward those who disobeyed, but kind to you if you continue to trust in His kindness. But if you stop trusting, you also will be cut off.

Romans 11:22

The living God is a very serious God. He desires to have a relationship with His creation, but must allow His crown of creation the choice of rejecting His grace. God has created this dynamic relationship of choice between His gifts of reconciliation or our own Ego centered self-controlled life. We have been given a choice between our Ego Self guiding our Path, or letting go and trusting the living God to take control of our Core & Path. The key to this whole transformation actually happens when we as humans *completely* die to ourselves and trust in His compassion to save us from ourselves.

> *Either way, Christ's love controls us. Since we believe that Christ died for all, we also believe that we have all died to our old life.*
>
> – 2 Corinthians 5:14 (NLT)

So when God comes into our spiritual being *(heart/soul)* and welds Himself to our True-Self, we are commissioned to use that unconditionally loving Holy Spirit's heart to melt the unbelieving hearts and the uncircumcised believing Christian hearts to be re-welded to the spiritual body of Christ. When His hot hand of Grace is on our hearts, it starts a melting process to soften our hearts for the divine welding process to begin. This is the evidence that God has started His wonderful process of transforming in us to a new creature predestined to be just like Him someday in Heaven for eternity.

"Your spiritual growth during this personal time of transformation will speak volumes about your heart for God and how your gifts and energy can impact the Kingdom of God. Those closest to you, family and long time friends will need time and space to appreciate and respect these transformational changes. The emotional baggage of your past still hangs around the corners of their perception of you, so you'll need patience and understanding with their learning curve. But I believe if you follow the protocol that God is unfolding in your life, there will be sustaining transformations they know not, because they're too close to the old you. If they truly care about you they will probably test the credibility of your commitment and grow to respect and give thanks as your past fades and the new transformed you shines to glorify God."

– Richard Cobb

Core Transformation Summary Points

- It is natural to fight reaching "the edge" – it's ok to have bad events to help you go to the edge so you can turn yourself over to God's Grace. A bad year in life is a good year for your soul.

- In the same way that an alcoholic has to accept that they are powerless over alcohol and that their lives have become completely unmanageable, those who are willing to allow true transformation of our Core must accept this same fact that we are powerless over sin.

- We must die this metaphorical death at our Core for the seeds of faith that have been planted through the miracle of birth and God's purification process of binding with our spiritual Core to start His reconciliation process. This transformation process of dying a metaphorical death is just like how a forest is reborn after a forest fire.

- Life's best pathways to the most marvelous transformations almost always come as a surprise! Remember, you can't invent your path to transformation because the Creator has the power to carve that path paired up with the grace to mercifully light the way He has planned for us.

Our job is to just walk in that light!

- Because God is love and filled with grace! It is only logical that God would give the crown of His creation one last chance before they die. But if you don't want to let go of your Ego-self and accept His saving grace even on our deathbed, God won't force you to save your soul.

- "If you follow the protocol that God is unfolding in your life, there will be sustaining transformations that some will not see, because they were too close to the "your old Self." And they will probably need to test the credibility of your new commitments and grow to respect and give thanks as the past fades and your new True Self shines to glorify God."

  Richard Cobb

- I believe God knows how hard it is to die to yourself and truly trust Him to be Lord of your life. He is patient and full of grace. God is always right there to save us from ourselves, even when sin has caused us to hide from His unconditional healing love.

- Don't try to invent the path for yourself. The Creator has a plan. He will carve the path for you and will grace you as you take on this endeavor. Open yourself up and trust the creator by walking into the light.

CHAPTER FOUR

Discovering Your Path

Your chosen Path is not outside of God's will. It will always be aligned with His master plan for His creation. So, seeking self-help processes instead of seeking alignment with God first is foolishness. Just control yourself on your path and live your life with a clear conscience. God will reveal your Path if you just trust His fatherly guidance.

We worry so much about what is ahead on our Path, instead of discovering our "Idiosyncratic Path" that will truly bring peace in our lives. We need to have faith and trust that what will unfold on our Path is good for our Core. God has already prepared the next phase of our life. We just need to let go and be happy and joyful, feeling blessed with the knowledge that God is in control.

I believe the biggest decision you will ever make at this critical point in your life; is choosing to discover your purpose filled Path or staying on the Path your ego driven mind thinks is best for you.

True Self is the Key to Discovery

This is the first step of finding your purpose filled Path. You can't even begin to find your right Path until your Core transformation has started. Your Ego-self must submit before your True Self can start to emerge. This typically happens after you have "Hit the Wall" and your Ego-self has failed you. We all need to accept the fact that we have ego driven human evil at our cores. Believing we are born pure and without sin is an egocentric lie. Because of Adam, the first sinner in the Garden of Eden, we are all natural born sinners. Every child is born with a strong Ego-self protecting Core. This is the part that has to submit and die to ourselves, so that your True Self, which was planted as a seed in your core while you were still in your mother's womb, can link with the living God.All we have to do is choose to open this spiritual door of our Core to Him so He can start the divine transformational process.

First the question is why is it important to have a path? It will give you peace and blessings. Peace that passes all understanding of the mind and blessings as defined in the original text as meaning "Enviably Happy." You might ask yourself, why would God the creator, want you to be "Enviably Happy?" Because this is how others will desire His process of reconciliation and peace in this world of un-fulfillment.

The True Self we discussed in the last chapter re-connecting with God the Creator who put the seed of your Core purpose in you before you were born; is the only part of the Core that can reveal your chosen Path and Life Purpose to your mind. As your True Self emerges from your core, your life purpose finally starts being revealed. Finding the right path and setting the right guiderails keeps alignment with your True Self and right Path.

In the next chapter I will reveal the guiderails God has created since the beginning of time that will help us lead this purpose driven life. Each person's path is idiosyncratic, which is why your right Path, is a narrow Path. In other words: each person's Path is special to himself or herself.

There is no one Path for everyone. Each person created is like a fingerprint. Every individual's Path is different. You cannot say, "This is the path of success for you" or "This is what you need to do to be a good Christian" or "If you follow my path you will be happy and prosperous."

You are created unique. You are not like everyone else. When people go to read a "how-to" book, it normally gets applied inappropriately as it might not align with your True Path. Most of these processes that people share for "self-help" are really targeted to your ego based mind. Aligning to this belief that happiness and success can be a packaged formula for everybody is like a diet. It doesn't work or last for most people.

So this is why discovering your Idiosyncratic Path is so critical. Because it was chosen for you as part of your spiritual genetic structure before you were born. Your True Path is not a straight path, the way our Ego Self would want it to be. That's what's so amazing! It is not straight, so your brain can't figure out your spiritual roadmap from point to point. Why did God make it so hard? Because without failure on your Path, your Ego Self starts to believe over time that you don't need anyone but yourself, not even God the restorer. When your sinful self brings you to the "Edge" or the "Wall" on this crazy Path called life, you can let go again and have faith in God controlling the outcome. Faith is built at your Core from letting go with your mind. Holding onto God's promises through tough times builds endurance. Endurance builds hope and hope builds faith as scripture says in Romans 5:4

Patient endurance develops maturity of character (approved faith and tried integrity). And character of this sort produces the habit of joyful and confident hope of eternal salvation.

Don't set out to find the Path to make your life easier. It's about being on the *"Right Path."* Don't assume everything bad that happens to you is necessarily bad for your Path. These things might be exactly what you need to keep you or get you back on your right Path. Many times what we think are knocking us off our Path is actually pushing us back on our chosen right Path.

It will become clearer that you have a predestined Life's Purpose for your Path. Your life's purpose is your rudder to hold yourself steady on your Path. If we yield to our True Self we will expose the light to our True Path. Remember I talked about turning your search light off. This helps your True Self see the True Path. Ego driven selfish desires will prevent you from seeing your chosen path. When you are trying to control the outcomes—the rings of your life, instead of following your GPS (God Positioning System)—it steers you off your chosen Path.

This whole issue about controlling outcomes in your *"Concentric Life Rings"* to try and make your Path what you think is right for you doesn't really work. Most of the outcomes will not turn out for you as you think they should. It is focusing on your alignment and restoration of your Core that you feel most comfortable and confident. You can't control other people or other situations to make your life easier. You can only control yourself. It's because everyone has their own path, even your children. We naturally impose our Path onto others we care about. True peace and the feeling of balance that we all search for is not found in outcomes. It's found in knowing you are on the *"Right Path"* with a clear conscience, founded in Hope and Trust in a power greater than ourselves. It's feeling at peace in the storm. When you are on your right path you will have a feeling of peace that your brain won't understand. God gives you a peace beyond your understanding. God gives you a peace that your brain will not ever understand.

Have you ever made a choice to do something that your cognitive understanding of the situation is in question, but your heart still feels that it is right?

So maybe it is better to lead with your heart (or True Self) in making major decisions. Leading physiologists will tell you that most people will think through all the data on a situation, and then make the decision with their gut feeling at the end.

As soon as you start managing your Path and start trying to control the outcomes in your life, you are not doing it in faith, are you? The key to your True Path is that you are allowing your Path to be revealed in faith and trust. It is very counter-intuitive to the brain and this world. How foolish can you be not controlling your own path? Don't you have any responsibility for your own life? But your true responsibility here is to trust your Life Purpose and Path that is being revealed to you as you move forward in this new life. Your True Path will be revealed to you. It is not something you build or search for.

This process is counter-intuitive to what we have been taught the way the world works. Faith is the key to unlocking your True Self and revealing your True Path. If you will truly let go of your Ego Self by listening and opening your inner eyes of your True Self, God will reveal your path. Trust Him!

> *"You will show me the path of life. In your presence is fullness of joy. At your right hand there are pleasures forever more."*
>
> Psalm 16:11

Light for, Barriers to and Signs on "Your Path"

The Light for Your Path

If we search for our Path with our Ego minds, our searchlight is too bright to see our chosen Path subtly lit by the Spirit of God. When we have the faith to shut off our minds by quietly trusting and listening from our True Self, we will start to see the path created for us. This process of letting go and trusting God will bring you happiness, pleasure and peace in your life. Then and only then will we be thankful for God's guidance and grace.

Barriers to Your Right Path

The first barriers are the mindsets in our culture and our own adaptive human development of our Ego Selves—not wanting to let go of control and allow God to start your Core transformation. The right Path is based in truth and can only be revealed to your True Self. Your Ego Self naturally searches for which path to take, but your True Self has the power of choice to allow your Path to be revealed without creating it. Relinquishing control of your Path to God is counter-intuitive to your mind. It will not seem logical to let go and trust God with your outcomes. It is risking the vulnerability of a child at your Core. The key is to stop looking for perfect choices to get desired outcomes on your Path.

Signs you are on the Right Path

It is important to know in your heart and mind that you are on this Right Path chosen by the Creator. Many people that are Ego-driven to a Path that they think will be right for them, find themselves disappointed with themselves and God. To insure that you are on your chosen Right Path, there will be signs that confirm it along the way. First is that you will have deep rooted passion about your Path and are normally moved to tears during the revelation of your Life Purpose and Right Path. It will feel right and also resonate deep in your Core.

Second, surprisingly, you won't have to force yourself to stay on the Right Path. You will have a connection to it that will go past your understanding. You will only be comfortable and at peace when you are on your Right Path.

If your Core and Path are aligned with your chosen Life Purpose, it should move you to rescue other broken people, and you will start to see the needs of others around you. It will change you from being rescued to rescuing others.

Follow God beyond self-control

If you follow God beyond what you can control, beyond where your own strengths and competencies can take you, beyond what is affirmed or considered a risk by the people around you, then you will experience God and His power, His wisdom and His love for you, more than you can ever imagine.

God is calling you to follow him to a place of weakness when you risk with the vulnerability of a child that you might know how strong your heavenly Father is and how much He loves you.

It's important that we respect this Path of faith by doing our part in having critical guiderails in place that help control ourselves, ensuring we stay "On Purpose." We have a responsibility to control ourselves. These aren't guardrails to *control* our Path or the outcomes on our Path.

Discovering Your Path Summary Points

- I believe the biggest decision you will ever make at this critical point in your life; is choosing to discover your purpose filled Path or staying on the Path your ego driven mind thinks is best for you.

- You can't even begin to find your purpose filled Path until your Core transformation has started. Your Ego-self must submit before your True Self can start to emerge. This typically happens after you have "Hit the Wall" and your Ego-self has failed you.

- If we search for our Path with our Ego centered minds, our searchlight is too bright to see our chosen Path subtly lit by the Spirit of God. When we have the faith to shut off our minds by quietly trusting and listening from our True Self, we will start to see the path created for us.

- The right Path is based in truth and can only be revealed to your True Self. Your Ego-Self naturally searches for which path to take, but your True Self has the power of choice to allow your Path to be revealed without creating it. Relinquishing control of your Path to God is counter-intuitive to world thought.

- Lead with your heart. Often your heart and gut trumps logic. True self is the key to Core discovery. Yield to it and the Light of Truth will reveal it to you.

- If your Core and Path are aligned with your chosen Life Purpose, it should move you to rescue other broken people, and you will start to see the needs of others around you. It will change you from being rescued to rescuing others.

- If you follow God beyond what you can control, beyond where your own strengths and competencies can take you, beyond what is affirmed or considered a risk by the people around you, then you will experience God and His power, His wisdom and His love for you, more than you can ever imagine. God is calling you to follow him to a place of weakness when you risk with the vulnerability of a child that you might know how strong your heavenly Father is and how much he loves you.

CHAPTER FIVE

Critical Guiderails

Guiderails are critical in this process of transformation. They provide the railings to keep you from straying off your new narrow Path as your life starts to speed up again. As your Core becomes transformed to a healthier state of heart & mind and all your Life Rings around you start engaging again, everything will start coming at you faster. When you start down your new Path the most important thing is the alignment between God's plan for you and your personal choices along your Path. Personal guiderails for your choices hold the key to finding peace at your Core and staying on the right Path in this world that seems to be falling apart all around us.

Guiderails are necessary within these key aspects of self:

- *Respecting your relationship with God*
- *Managing the desires of this world*
- *Growth of character*
- *Personal disciplines*
- *Spiritual growth*
- *Physical health*
- *Daily decision making*
- *Major path decisions*

What I am going to share with you in this chapter are the major foundational guiderails. They will not come as a surprise, but I hope the words describing them will bless you and give you the desire to use them with wisdom.

There is a critical reason for putting these in place. God's Word contains the guiderails to keep you on the right Path; also to keep you focused on your new narrow Path. The perfect timing of good outcomes tends to unfold slower than we, in this Ego driven fast paced world, think it should. God knows how to use time for more than one micro purpose.

Your Ego-Self naturally searches for which path to take, but your True Self has the power to allow your Path to be revealed without creating it. Relinquishing control of your Path to God is counter-intuitive, but you can trust His timing of outcomes are perfect and always has a positive ripple effect on future generations. He directs things to slow down and align allowing more hearts to line up at the same time having a positive ripple effect.

We naturally try to control the outcomes in our Life Rings, but what we should be controlling is our Ego Self, which has the power to cause conflict and damage for us in our Life Rings. We should stay away from unhealthy relationships that divert us from our Right Path. Unhealthy relationships tend to not be reciprocal in benefit for both parties and the outcomes normally benefit only one side of the relationship. Having relationships in your life that are based on only giving or taking will cause damage to your True Self, and bring out your Ego Self to protect your Core by trying to control the outcomes in your life.

Reciprocal signs on your Path will show up when your relationships are healthy. You normally get back from others what you give out. Old friends and new friends will come into your Life Rings directed by the Spirit to help confirm what God is teaching you. Others will confirm your transformational changes and see the work that God is doing in your life.

If you are attempting to control the major outcomes in your Life Rings during this transformational process, it will not bring you happiness and peace. Trying to control the people around you will only bring you conflict and frustration, not happiness. Also, thinking that bad situations are taking you off your path is just your Ego Self not being satisfied but in reality they might be bringing you back on to your chosen Path.

Being Honest with your Self is a critical Guiderail!

May our conscience testify that we have conducted ourselves in obedience and honesty that comes from God, not in human wisdom, but from the Grace of God, especially in our relationships with others!

Romans 12 sheds some light on some behaviors that will start to emerge after a true transformation. Such as no longer modeling our lives after the customs of the world, but rather, letting God transform you into a new person by changing the way you think. You now will learn to know God's voice directing your new Path, which will be pleasing and perfect.

It is important that you never think you are better than you really are. Be honest in your evaluation of yourself, measuring yourselves by the faith God has given you. Don't pretend to love others. Really love them. Hate what is wrong. Hold tightly to what is good and fair in everyone's sight. Love each other with genuine affection and respect, taking delight in honoring each other. Never pay back evil with more evil. Do things in such a way that allows everyone to see you are honorable and kind. Strive to live in peace with everyone. Never take revenge, leave it to the righteous anger of God. For the scripture says:

"I will take revenge; I will pay them back," says the Lord!

Value Benchmarks

There are ten value benchmarks as guiderails:

1. *Truth telling – for a clear conscience*
2. *Small incremental steps – for true transformation*
3. *Justly measured grace – balance between kindness and tough love*
4. *Empathy in action – forgiveness sets you free*
5. *Unearned compassion – "paying it forward"*
6. *Doing the "next right thing" – a heart of obedience*
7. *Integrity – <u>Being</u> the right person to start <u>Doing</u> the right things*
8. *Confirmation fruit – evidence that you are on the right path*
9. *Lead by example – actions do speak louder than words*
10. *Living your chosen path – life changing*

Core Values

We should hold the same Core Values that God reflects in His personality if He is now truly living in us through transformation of the Core.

Here are seven Core Values:

1. Truth
2. Forgiveness
3. Respect
4. Righteousness
5. Faithfulness
6. Kindness
7. Love

Truth

The Truth will set you free—Truth about yourself will set you free to follow God's plan for your life. Freedom can't be forced because God respects your freedom of choice. Because Jesus was the son of man and the son of God, He is the Truth that sets you free from the bondage of yourself. Truth about yourself is essential to discovering your True Self at your Core. Your Ego Self will try and block you from accepting the Truth about yourself. Only the Holy Spirit of Truth can "prick the heart" to accept that we are evil and need rescuing by the Creator God. Truth will replace faith completely because when time in this world comes to an end, only Truth will exist since nothing will ever change again. So where is Truth? Truth is in you. God wants you to live in Truth with Him. You need to be Truthful to others, to God and most of all to yourself. God is a just God and must judge all things, or He could not hold all Truth.

God is the mirror and scale of our hearts

"TEKEL" — you have been weighed on the scales and found deficient.

Daniel 5:27

Small lies wipe out a great deal of Truth. Hebrews 14 says nothing in all creation is hidden from God. He is the one to whom we are all accountable.

Forgiveness

Forgiveness gives up the right to accuse others for hurting you. It sets you free to follow your new Path. Forgiveness is like love: it's a choice that you make. As you truly forgive others it releases your anger and allows God's grace to enter your life. When you forgive people you start liking yourself more, freeing you to give more to others without needing acceptance or expecting anything in return. Any time you give of yourself to others, your ego feels the need to get something back from them. If someone in your life convinces your Ego Self that you're responsible for their unhappiness in this life, you end up not loving yourself; which is why we have a hard time loving others unconditionally. For example if you tell a child that she or he is a bad child for enough years, they will see themselves as a bad person. If you tell them enough times they are a good child, they will see themselves as a good person. We are very impressionable humans and believe almost anything that people say about us. Whenever you accept that God loves you just the way you are, then you can start to accept and love others unconditionally.

Whatever emotional needs you feel are lacking from your life partner relationship like:

- ***Admiration***
- ***Affection***
- ***Appreciation***
- ***Commitment***
- ***Financial Needs***
- ***Open & Honest Conversation***
- ***Physical Attractiveness***
- ***Recreational Companionship***
- ***Respect***
- ***Sexual Fulfillment***
- ***Trust***

You will get them filled from someone else: family, children, friends, co-workers and even strangers. If someone truly believes that your love for them is so strong that whatever they do, you will still love them and forgive them; this is God's unconditional Grace flowing though you. This allows the receiver the freedom to be open and honest with their personal struggle with sin and removes the deception that their sin has damaged the love from the unconditional (Agape') lover. Forgiveness gives us the power to be open and honest, living our life in the light of truth. Nothing is more powerful than the power of forgiving someone of an unforgivable action or word. People that we let into our lives affect our Cores each day. That's why it is so important that as you start your new life, you become more selective with the people you spend the majority of your time with.

The giving of an undeserved gift of forgiveness at the right time to people that you feel have hurt you releases you and exposes them to God's grace.

Forgiveness does not create a relationship but without it you cannot sustain a healthy relationship. A trusting relationship can only be established again, if both parties are open, honest and truthful about what caused the conflict. Although conflict is the foundation of a good relationship if it is resolved before damage is done at a core level. Most people believe the myth that if you have conflict, you don't have a good relationship. But these are the things that bring us together. The restoration of a relationship where a sinful behavior has caused conflict with two parties is just the process God has created for redeeming the crown of His creation. God created conflict when He created choice and the concept of "good & evil." Each part has a purpose. If the law was not created, sin would have no power to condemn us. For the world, Christ was like a seed that was buried and then rose again in new growth. That conflict was the door that opened to the resolution of God reconciling His creation.

Forgiveness through *kindness and unconditional love* are the only things that bring people to repent. True repentance through transformation of the heart & mind is required for a foundation of trust to rebuild any relationship. If you don't truly repent allowing the transformation of the heart and mind to begin,

God's grace can not do the work to forgive you and rebuild the relationship with Him.

Repentance is a change of ones mind for the better, heartily amending ones ways, with abhorrence of His past sins, in order to obtain forgiveness of and release from your sinful self.

Unforgiving people have long memories. They don't let go. Some people can hold a grudge for a lifetime. Love never keeps a record of another's offenses. There is an Eskimo word for forgiveness: ***(Issumagijoujungnainermik)*** meaning you are not thinking about it anymore. Forgiveness sometimes is more powerful for the one forgiving than the person that causes the pain. When someone hurts you they typically don't think about it for very long, but you can carry that pain for a lifetime.

"Forgive us our sins as we forgive those who sin against us"

God has taught us directly through Jesus in the *"Lords Prayer" Matthew 6:12,* that He will forgive us our sins as we forgive those that have hurt us with their sin.

Respect

Respect is the cornerstone of every healthy relationship. In every relationship if there is not a reciprocal balance of respect, growth won't occur. Whether it's a teacher-student, parent-child, boss-employee, spouses, friends, you and God, or even the relationship between humans and pets, the need for respect as the foundation for a good relationship is critical.

You can find yourself in love with someone you don't Respect, but you can't stay in love them.

We also need to Respect our True Selves and if we do, we start to Respect our body and our soul and our minds. This guiderail helps us appreciate and honor our chosen Path. Respecting the feelings of those who trust and love us, as well as respecting others whose Cores and Paths we affect each day.

We need to Respect God's requirements for a relationship with the Creator. The hardest thing to go through is when God starts blessing you with the pleasures of this world. It is so easy to get caught up in activity managing and consuming your time with good things in your life that you forget to spend the time alone with He who rescued you after "Hitting the Wall." God is just like our earthly fathers in how He wants to give us what we desire—as long as we can stay humble, thankful, and respectful of our relationship with Him and others.

Righteousness

"The Lord has told you what is good and this is what He requires of you—to do what is right, to love mercy and to walk humbly with your God."

Micah 6:8 NLT

What does it mean to "do what's right?" There is a difference between figuring out what is right that will give us the results we desire for our future, along with trying to do the right things to please God; vs. accepting the truth that we only have the power to do the "next right thing" with God's direction through His Word and Spiritual guidance. In making that choice you find that you have both "Sides of Self" influencing your decision. With every major choice you make, both your Ego Self and your True Self are influencing you.

This conflict at your Core makes each choice no matter how big or small critical in your Core development.

God desires to guide us. He desires that we are righteous like Him. Scripture says we are pre-destined to be like Him. When you accept God into your Core, you are pre-destined to be like His son that was Flesh and God's Spirit combined. Doing the right thing like the saying "What Would Jesus Do," is letting go and trusting that the choices you are making are directed and confirmed by Him.

You need to respect and trust the power of God's mercy. Righteousness is a *gift* of mercy. God's Grace is founded in unconditional Love (Agape'). There is nothing we can do to earn it no matter how good we become in our own eyes and others around us. We should encourage others to forgive and to love mercy also. If you accept that God has forgiven your human evil state of being, then your True-Self can walk humbly with God. Righteousness cannot be achieved by trying to please God with our actions, because our righteousness is filthy rags in God's eyes. It's about God being righteous through us each day. All we can do is get out of the way and let Him lead our lives through faith in the promises He has made us.

It's about your Core being at the right place with God. Being the right person at your Core is the only way to start doing the right things. It's about being humble and faithful. It is having the faith of Abraham, the father of our faith that will please God, not doing the right things. The only thing that is counted as righteousness in heaven is your faith in God's promises.

> *For the Scriptures tell us, "Abraham believed God, and God counted him as righteous because of his faith."*
>
> Romans 4:3 NLT

Many religions teach people's minds to control their sinful lives and thoughts, all to no avail, because our righteousness will always fall short of God's expectations. These teachings actually keep us from the edge, while all the time God is trying to bring you to the edge—the wall of breakthrough, letting go and trusting Him in faith.

God needs us to stay humble to do His work through us. It's about embracing failure, embracing we are sinful, embracing the edge. It's about the Holy Spirit taking us to the edge through our choices and God wanting to forgive us and ultimately rescue us from our sinful selves.

Righteousness as a guiderail is God working through us to keep His promises, not us becoming more righteous. Remember this is a process, not a one time fix. This process will repeat for the rest of our lives if we continue to "Let go" and trust Him. This book should be helping expose your Core with the light of counter-intuitive truth, allowing you to begin discovering your own unique Path. We are all uniquely special in God's master plan that has accounted for every detail in creation.

There will be many false Messiahs and Prophets imitating Christ, saying, "Follow my Path!" But your Path is Idiosyncratic to you alone, amazingly unique like your fingerprint. That's the mystery and beauty of God's comprehensive ability to create over a hundred billion unique humans as the crown of His creation. There is only one righteous entity or power in the universe, which is God Himself. The Almighty God will reveal Himself to you with your own unique personal relationship with Him. Once the living God, by power of the risen Christ has spiritually bonded with your True Self, you are predestined to have Him take more space in your Core, so the Ego-self has to diminish.

Therefore your righteousness is the seed of faith that God has placed in your Core with His Spirit. God sees our hearts before we act. So if we are right in our heart, we are right with God. There are many people who think they can innocently desire, but as long as they don't act on it, they are right with themselves and God, but they're not. Being right means you feel and know you are right in your heart instead of just *controlling* what you do to appear right to God and others. When humans believe they can entertain sinful thoughts in their mind and heart and still feel justified because they don't act it out, they become hypocritical of others. You start to become a judge of other people's behavior to make yourself feel better at your Core. It's not about God's mercy anymore. Instead, it is all about controlling your façade.

This is not righteousness. It is self-righteousness!

Being right with God is about spending one-on-one time with Him—listening rather than just talking to Him. You can call it prayer time, meditation time, but it is one-on-one time with the Creator. God makes us righteous by taking a place in our Core and shutting our minds and egos down, so He can communicate with our True Selves and through transformation change the way we think. I am hoping by now you're getting the point that as a guiderail it is not about human righteousness.

There is only one righteous and it is God.

Faithfulness

Just like a lot of this book is counter-intuitive to the way our ego self has been developed to protect us or we have been taught through education and religion that faithfulness is for the benefit of the receiver. Most of the time it is not noticed or appreciated by the receiver! God does not need our faithfulness; but wants us to be faithful like He is faithful.

Faithfulness bears good fruit in the life of the one being faithful. We have been raised to believe that being unfaithful hurts others more than ourselves. This is a deception by our Ego. It eats at your Core for the rest of your life. Unfaithfulness feeds the development of our Ego Self and diminishes our True Selves. So the real problem is that when we are only faithful to ourselves in situations, being unfaithful to others for our own ego self-protection; it destroys our self-esteem and reduces our self worth.

God must be faithful even if we are not, because that is who He is. Our ego wants us to believe being faithful is a benefit to others. This is why it is so easy to lie. You are lying essentially to be faithful, so as to protect others from the truth. Faithfulness is of the heart, not just actions. If you think about situations of unfaithfulness but don't act on those thoughts, you are still unfaithful. It's about what is in your heart. It's about you being honest with your True Self and God.

Jesus knew what they were thinking, so He asked them, "Why do you have such evil thoughts in your hearts?"

Matthew 9:4

"You have heard the commandment that says, 'You must not commit adultery.' But I say, anyone who even looks at a woman with lust has already committed adultery with her in his heart."

Matthew 5:27-28

We should be faithful in all things and to others because it allows our hearts and souls to live in peace. Do all things in full faith and don't judge yourself according to how much faith others have. What's counter-intuitive to the brain is that we have been trained in our minds that faithfulness is hard: That faithfulness is a duty. The fruit of faithfulness is acceptance and trust from others. Unfaithfulness destroys your life more so than even the life of others. Others recover from your unfaithfulness faster than your Core does. It's like having cancer of the Core. Also, if you don't go through God's process of transformation the guilt and shame of being unfaithful stays with you forever.

The damage you can do to your own Core by being unfaithful could be eternal!

If you really do care about yourself and you love yourself, you will be faithful—to others, to God and to yourself—in your actions, heart and mind. God sees our heart every second of every day. For me, God loved me enough to take me through His process of facing my unfaithfulness.

Going through the process, God directed me to a book titled "Respectable Sins." What I now understand is that all sins that cause damage in our lives and others start out in our hearts and minds as small seeds to protect our ego. These sins are acceptable in most cultures and most religions. Occasionally we create little white lies to deal with uncomfortable situations. We do this because our ego self tells us we have the right to manipulate the truth because we are protecting the ones we are lying to. I now see that this is more damaging than telling the people the truth. We call these white lies like we have the power to judge how to divide the truth. When you tell the truth, people are more willing to help you get through the problem. Humans hate to be lied to.

In our society people feel if you don't lie you are not "up to par" with others and will be taken advantage of. The unspoken truth in our society is that everyone is unfaithful. It's easy to judge others when you think you are right, because you are controlling some of your actions. We are all unfaithful in our hearts and minds. God set up these rules to condemn us by making these Laws impossible to meet. Otherwise we would not need Him to save us from ourselves.

It says in the Bible that if just one person could have kept the Law, Christ would have died in vain. Because of Adam's sin of unfaithfulness we are all sinners. The deception is that we can achieve acceptance from God by doing the right things in life. What we must come to grips with is the truth that we are all unfaithful and fall short of the glory of God no matter what level of perceived spiritual enlightenment we achieve. If we try with our own ego to be faithful, so others will accept us, we will fail. We can only be faithful by letting go of our Ego-Self and let God transform us to be like Him. God is faithful!

There was a woman I met with whom I shared what God was doing in my life. The next week she contacted me to tell me her story of relationships. Her husband who she loved dearly had died a few years back and left her with over a million dollars in debt and was forced to file bankruptcy. She thought they were financially comfortable for the rest of their lives. While he was fighting brain cancer, he started to make bad investment decisions. Her husband didn't want her to know the dire financial situation they were getting into. He thought he was protecting her from the truth, so she wouldn't worry and she blindly trusted him with her security.

Years after he a had passed away and she was working her way back out of debt she had found a new guy that she loved and he gave her a feeling of solid financial security and a new fresh start. He had convinced her to quit her job and he would support her until she got her real estate business up and going. Days after we met through a mutual friend she ended up contacting me from a hospital where she was visiting him, only to discover he also had a life-threatening situation similar to her last husband. That day she went to withdraw money from her ATM account and found that it was overdrawn. She asked him in the hospital to tell her the truth about their financial situation, and he then said there is no more money. He was worried if she found out she would leave him, so until that day he was hiding the truth from her. She found herself in the exact same situation all over again and felt like she was going to lose her mind, trying to understand why this is happening to her again.

Deceitful perception management to hold a relationship together, instead of exposing the truth to your partner and trying to work it out together, erodes the strongest relationships. This deception mindset to hold onto love is becoming more common in our culture, as we continue to slide into this world where the cultural foundations of our past are crumbling. One of the most damaging actions to someone you love is lying to them, believing your protecting them from the painful truth of a situation. Also trusting in any person with blind faith becomes the catalyst of unfaithfulness in our relationships. Child like should be reserved for our relationship with God. So being open and honest in our relationships is a critical guiderail if we ever want to be happy.

Humans will lie to us about God, but God will never lie to us. He is truth!

Kindness

There are some people that think just by being quiet and patient they are being kind. This is not necessarily true; their motivation can be to avoid conflict with others. So you can be patient and endure abuse from someone without response to avoid more unkindness to you. But by not responding, you fantasize that you will be okay and the person will stop harassing you. In most cases the abuse doesn't goes away. It will typically come back another day. If someone is abusing you—physically or emotionally—and you don't say anything, you force yourself to believe that you are helping that relationship. It is the same situation whether they are your spouse, parent, child, boss, bully or terrorist. *You need to be proactive!*

Kindness is:

- *Pro-active versus patient*
- *Serving others graciously*
- *Giving without thinking*
- *Being humble when others are not*
- *Communicating compassion or doing something for others*
- *Enduring abuse without a defensive response*
- *Repaying evil with good deeds*
- *Seeing the good in all things*
- *An unconditional action of the heart*
- *Not looking for a reciprocal action*

There is a scripture in the Bible that states that if you are kind to someone who is bad to you it is like putting hot coals on their forehead. Undeserving kindness is founded in unconditional love. Kindness is something you can give. It is a choice just like love. Being proactively kind allows the light of God's Grace to penetrate someone's ego-protected Core, allowing their humble True Self to emerge so God's Grace can start the transformation process of their hearts hardened by life.

Kindness has the power to reach into someone's Core to begin a change of heart

Don't you see how wonderfully kind, tolerant, and patient God is with you? Does this mean nothing to you? Can't you see that His kindness is intended to turn you from your sin?

Romans 2:3-5 NLT

His grace provides the guiderails that through *being kind* allows the light of Truth and the warmth of His Grace into this dark cold world.

The point is not the exposure of right and wrong. Or finding out what you need to do to make your Core right with God. It's about exposing your Core to the Light of Truth. God's *kindness* will allow this to happen painlessly. God loves to forgive and restore. As the old saying goes, love is patient and kind. Christ said, "Trust me and I will show you my kindness," He has to be kind just as He has to be faithful. That's who God is. That's what Agape' love is; undeserving kindness. Christ died for our sins *before* we committed them. That's what being the true Messiah is about.

Never let loyalty and kindness leave you! Tie them around your neck as a reminder. Write them deep within your heart.

Proverbs 3:2-4 NLT

Love

Love has so much power. We just don't know how to use it!

The most interesting thing about Love is that it is the strongest emotion in the universe; it has power over fear, unfaithfulness and human evil. This makes Love the most critical of all the guiderails. It is an emotion, but until it is turned into action it has little affect. Love is a choice, not just a feeling. People think that they can find love by falling into it or they need to find someone that's the perfect partner, so that they can love them. You can love people who don't love you or don't even know who you are. It's your choice!

God loved His creation so much that He made a choice to give of Himself in the form of a human being, feeling the temptation of sin that He created, but having the power not to yield to the power of sin. This made Him the only perfect sacrifice to redeem creation for the consequence of sin which is death. As a result, Christ had to die when He took on the sins of the world.

Because God took the consequence for sin to the grave for Love, it allowed the Holy Spirit to enter into a human Core, but only through Faith and Hope.

This process of reconciliation cannot happen by doing good deeds or meeting the expectation of the Law in any way. This is how God loved us before we were born and before we were transformed having His Spirit in our Cores. When we accept God into our Core, we then have a piece of God (Christ) in us and we become children of God in His eyes. Then He will not just Love you, but start raising you like His only child to be just like Him for eternity, so our spirits can enjoy spending eternity with Him with no end.

God is love at His core. He doesn't just "do" love, He "is" love.

What is true love? Actions are more powerful than words: humility, obedience to your commitments, and self-sacrifices for others, meeting needs of others and loving to the end. Love does not need to be loved back. We only have one word for Love in the English language; there are three words for Love in the Greek language. The Love you have just been reading about is Agage' love which means to love unconditionally. This type of love can only come from God and be channeled through us to others. I don't believe humans have the power in themselves without God to honestly love this way. The second kind of Love is Eros love; this is emotional and sensual love between human beings. This love was designed by God to be shared between just two people, one man and one woman. The third type of Love is Philo love, known as brotherly and sisterly love between friends and strangers.

Love cannot co-exist with self-centered anger. If there is a presence of selfish anger, honest love will be absent. You can be angry about something for the protection of others and still love, but you can't be angry defending yourself and still honestly love. If you truly love someone they will not be able to provoke you to be hurtful with your words. Love is also not given to any sudden outbursts of emotion or action which is ego driven.

So if we are in a state of love we will not have emotional outbursts. There are times in our lives when there are psychological reasons of chemical imbalance that affect our brains that can cause emotional outbursts. That's the exception.

If you believe that you don't need help with your thoughts or your righteousness, you actually don't love yourself enough to allow the truth to expose your human evil based condition. The only people that psychologist can't help are people that believe they don't need help. This is normally the case with people that scapegoat the responsibility for their own unhappiness.

If you truly love you are not emotionally affected by personal attacks. Love will actually confront the sin, but will accept the sinner at the same time. So many people will reject the sinner for their sinful behavior, and lose the opportunity to help the sinner at the time when sin has done its divine work of taking that person to the edge. That is when they need your love the most!

God came into this world driven by LOVE in the form of Jesus to forgive the people that know they are sinners not the people that think they're spiritually healthy. Hypocrites in their minds believe they are right and others are wrong. This type of mindset cannot be helped by anyone, except maybe God and the Divine process of allowing your Ego-self to take you to the edge.

Love exalts others while pride exalts our ego self. Love has the power to transform selfish people into unconditional givers. That's why only love and kindness will bring people to repentance and a change of behavior, not confronting them with truth about their sin or how evil or bad they are; they already know this in their hearts. This only makes them defend their sinful position and protect their Ego Self from narcissistic damage. Love and kindness will maybe help them "let go and let God" help them save them from themselves.

We must choose to love because it's not natural for us to love unconditionally. It is natural for us to protect ourselves. In fact, loving someone unconditionally is counter-intuitive to our own self-preservation.

This is not a choice for God. True Love forgives until it's not thought about any more. Real love won't remember being hurt. Love never justifies sin. It never compromises God's word. It always expects the best from others. And the most important thing love does is that it keeps spiritual insight from distortion, because spiritual insight without love makes people do evil things in the name of the Almighty God.

We can't create Love! All we can do is channel Love, because God is Love.

Critical Guiderails Summary Points

- Guiderails keep you from straying off your new narrow Path as your life starts to speed up again. As your Core becomes transformed to a healthier state of heart & mind and all your Life Rings around you start engaging again, everything will start coming at you faster.

- Unhealthy relationships tend to not be reciprocal in benefit for both parties and the outcomes normally benefit only one side of the relationship. Relationships in your life that are based on giving or taking will cause damage to your True Self, and bring out your Ego Self to protect your Core by trying to control outcomes in your life.

- The seven Core values as guiderails on your new path are Truth, Forgiveness, Respect, Righteousness, Faithfulness, Kindness and Love.

- Small lies wipe out a great deal of Truth. Hebrews 14 says nothing in all creation is hidden from God. He is the one to whom we are all accountable.

- Many religions teach people's minds to control their sinful lives and thoughts, all to no avail, because our righteousness is like filthy rags in God's eyes. These teachings actually keep us from the edge, while all the time God is trying to bring you to the wall—the wall of breakthrough, letting go and trusting Him in faith.

- God must be faithful even if we are not, because that is who He is. Our ego wants us to believe being faithful is a benefit to others. This is why it is so easy to lie. You are lying essentially to be faithful, so as to protect others from the truth. Faithfulness is of the heart, not just actions. If you think about situations of unfaithfulness but don't act on those thoughts, you are still unfaithful. It's about what is in your heart. It's about you being honest with your True Self and God.

- Kindness is: Pro-active versus patient, Serving others graciously, Giving without thinking, Being humble when others are not, Communicating compassion or doing something for others, Enduring abuse without a defensive response, Repaying evil with good deeds, Seeing the good in all things, An unconditional action of the heart, Not looking for a reciprocal action.

- We must choose to love because it's not natural for us to love unconditionally. It is natural for us to protect ourselves. In fact, loving someone unconditionally is counter-intuitive to our own self-preservation.

- Love does not need to be loved back. We only have one word for Love in the English language; there are three words for Love in the Greek language. The Love you have just been reading about is Agage' love which means to love unconditionally. This type of love can only come from God and be channeled through us to others.

CHAPTER SIX

Failure & Faith

I chose to use the word "failure" because it is not just about making mistakes or sinning. It's about accepting the failure of our ego-driven choices. Once we accept failure we can start to have real faith. It's impossible to have faith when you "think" you can figure out the solution yourself. The cornerstone of failure comes from our own natural human evil. Roman 7 on the next page talks about God's law *revealing* our sin. Evil has a divine purpose to bring us condemned before God so He can reconcile us. Sin makes us feel like God has abandoned us in the same way Jesus felt as He was dying on the cross. He took on the sins of the world that *separated* the creation from the Creator. God NEVER leaves us. He never left Jesus abandoned on the cross. Christ felt that way because He took on the sins of the world separating Him from Adonai *(God the Father).*

> *When we were controlled by our old nature, sinful desires were at work within us, and the law aroused these evil desires that produced a harvest of sinful deeds, resulting in death. But now we have been released from the law, for we died to it and are no longer captive to its power. Now we can serve God, not in the old way of obeying the letter of the law, but in the new way of living in the Spirit. Did the law, which is good, cause my death? Of course not! Sin used what was good to bring about my condemnation to death. So we can see how terrible sin really is. It uses God's good commands for its own evil purposes. So the trouble is not with the law, for it is spiritual and good. The trouble is with me, for I am all too human, a slave to sin. I don't really understand myself, for I want to do what is right, but I don't do it. Instead, I do what I hate.*
>
> Romans 7:5-15 NLT

Natural Human Evil

Once evil gets exposed to the truth of what it really is, it loses its power. Once the light of truth exposes Satan, it reveals he has no power that God has not allowed. He is just a puppet of God's plan to bring us to the edge. We are all natural born sinners defending and preserving the integrity of our own ego developed sinful selves. In short it's scapegoating. For example we can accuse people that we have emotionally beaten down over time so we can use the power of blaming them for our own Core sinful issues, leaving them lacking the emotional power to escape from the relationship. This is displacing facing your own Core problems with blaming others for your unhappiness, because your Ego-Self is not willing to deal with your own Core issues.

Natural human evil minds believe that there is nothing wrong with their Core and they feel no need to "let go" and die to themselves. This is why most people feel they don't need faith. They think they have figured it all out. They are "ok." In a way *"evil"* is a personality disorder. The first behavior you will notice is a consistent scapegoating behavior that is very subtle in people that believe the deceptive evil lie that they are good at the Core. Second, they are very intolerant to criticism of any type that could be damaging to their narcissism. Third, there is a high concern for their self-image. They want to be respected and seen as stable and right by everyone around them. They are in denial of having any vengeful feelings or motives. Fourth, there is a certain intellectual deviousness that, at times, shows a disintegration of logic when they are under stress. Turning to God through faith alone, saving them from their failures is the only way for transformation.

Evil is defined as the use of power to destroy the spiritual growth of others for the sole purpose of defending and preserving their own narcissistic illness. People who hold on to this evil position deny the suffering of their guilt. They don't accept the painful awareness of their sin or their inadequacy and the damage that is caused by their own failures. They project their pain onto others through scapegoating.

To understand this concept in depth read "People of the Lie" by M. Scott Peck, M.D.

Endurance through Discipline

As you endure God's discipline (nobody likes it) you have to remember that God is treating you as His own child and what good parent doesn't discipline their child? If God doesn't discipline you as He does all of His children, it means you are an illegitimate child of God. *God is the author of tough love!*

> *And have you forgotten the encouraging words God spoke to you as his children? He said, "My child, don't make light of the* LORD*'s discipline, and don't give up when He corrects you. For the* LORD *disciplines those He loves, and He punishes each one He accepts as His child." As you endure this divine discipline, remember that God is treating you as His own children. Who ever heard of a child who is never disciplined by its father? If God does not discipline you as He does all of His children, it means that you are illegitimate and are not really His children at all. Since we respected our earthly fathers who disciplined us, shouldn't we submit even more to the discipline of the Father of our spirits, and live forever? For our earthly fathers disciplined us for a few years, doing the best they knew how. But God's discipline is always good for us, so that we might share in His Holiness. No discipline is enjoyable while it is happening—it's painful! But afterward there will be a peaceful harvest of right living for those who are trained in this way.*
>
> Hebrews 12:5-11 NLT

Since we respect our earthly father who has disciplined us, shouldn't we respect the discipline of God the Father of our spirit?

No discipline is ever enjoyable while it is happening but after, there is a good fruitful harvest from right doing. The result of this process is that *faith* is produced along with *endurance* and *trust* in the one who disciplines you. These are the "good fruits" of Failure.

> *We can rejoice, too, when we run into problems and trials, for we know that they help us develop endurance. And endurance develops strength of character, and character strengthens our confident hope of salvation. And this hope will not lead to disappointment. For we know how dearly God loves us, because He has given us the Holy Spirit to fill our hearts with His love.*
>
> Romans 5:3-5 NLT

Just like removing light for darkness to exist. You can't create darkness: it only exists when light is not there. Similarly, you can't make cold. An air conditioner removes heat so cold can exist. Whenever and wherever God removes His Spirit, evil will exist. So God does not do evil, but He has created the space for it to exist by removing His Spirit. This process that God created gave His creation choice between good and evil; the effect is that His creation is subjected to change.

When we sin we are blocking the awareness of God's presence in our lives, even though He has never left us. We feel like He has abandoned us, just like Jesus felt on the cross when He took on the sins of the world. God always uses evil for good over time: both in your daily life and in His master plan for all of creation. Evil has no power that God does not allow; all to fulfill His Devine purpose. He allows evil to do its work bring people and this planet to the edge or the wall. This process brings His creation to failure and in some cases through letting go and only trusting Him to save us from ourselves can God reconcile His creation back to Himself through Faith.

> *This Good News tells us how God makes us right in his sight. This is accomplished from start to finish by faith. As the Scriptures say, "It is through faith that a righteous person has life."*
>
> Romans 1:17 NLT

It's about letting God's Spirit guide us through a childlike faith and trust in a relationship with a personal caring father. You can't seem to tap into true pure faith until you "Hit the Wall" and fail from trying to manage our lives our way. Without failure there is no true need for faith. Understanding and accepting our failures allows our faith in a higher power to grow, allowing us to trust God with our future.

We should let sin and the Law do the work of condemning us as they were designed to do, keeping us humble through failure, so faith in God's promises are the only justification of hope in ever pleasing God. This is God's wonderful process of reconciliation.

If you take a hard look at what the areas are of importance for fulfillment in your life—how fulfilled are you in your career, your Kingdom work, your finances, your health, your relationships, your family, your life partner and your personal growth, you will start to see and understand what the areas could be for growth. Are you enjoying life? What would it take for you to be fulfilled today? To give you peace and a feeling of purpose that you are on your chosen Path.

Fulfillment is about your choices aligning with your core values, but it is not your effort of controlling outcomes for future fulfillment. It is just an illusion that we can capture fulfillment in the future. Our future never turns out the way we think!

Romantic relationships, friendships, business success, etc. are just expressions of fulfillment. They are not fulfillment itself. Fulfillment is the state of expressing who you really are, being the right person at your Core. It's about being fully alive. It's a feeling of wholeness, satisfaction, peace, rightness and harmony with the Creator; that can only happen through Failure and Faith.

Faith and Intelligence

Intelligence can only take you to the edge of all knowledge revealed so far in this world and then Faith has to be there to carry you to total truth. The knowledge of truth has an end to what we understand, but faith has no end while we are still in this world. When "time" comes to an end, everything will stop changing. When we get to heaven only truth will exist; Faith will no longer have a Devine purpose. Your mind can take you to the Edge; but you need Faith to break through the limits of your mind. You will never find certainty through an intellectual life, because it will only take you to the edge of knowledge.

Real faith will not grow until you let go and trust in a power other than yourself. You won't truly "let go" until you fail at doing your best trying to control the outcomes in your life. If you use your mind for a desired outcome to do something for a desired outcome, or try to influence outcomes to turn out the way you want, thinking it will work out for you or the ones you love; you don't need faith or trust in any power but your own.

As long as you are feeling successful in your efforts, you won't tap into real faith. Your mind will not let go until you "hit the wall" and accept failure at some level. That's why sin and the Mosaic Law were designed to condemn us and take us to the edge; but do nothing to save us or redeem us.

Eastern religions, including western Christianity like most religions, work hard to keep their followers from the edge or "hitting the wall." They teach us how to do the right things to please God. This is a problem because you can't do the right things to be the right person in God's eyes, but you can be the right person at your Core through transformation, so you start becoming like Christ which is the only way you can please the Living God. You must have God himself in you to be accepted by Him. Most religions don't teach you to "let go" of trying to please God by our own efforts. The truth is that you need to accept that you are a natural born sinner, before God's grace can do its divine purpose and rescue you. It is about a life on the other side of your Ego-self. The key is to accept in our heart and mind that it's OK to fail at God's tests; so we can humbly grow in faith and appreciate His powerful grace.

The Apostle Paul says, God's Law Reveals Our Sin

7 *Well then, am I suggesting that the law of God is sinful? Of course not! In fact, it was the law that showed me my sin. I would never have known that coveting is wrong if the law had not said, "You must not covet."*

8 *But sin used this command to arouse all kinds of covetous desires within me! If there were no law, sin would not have that power.*

9 *At one time I lived without understanding the law. But when I learned the command not to covet, for instance, the power of sin came to life,*

10 *and I died. So I discovered that the law's commands, which were supposed to bring life, brought spiritual death instead.*

11 *Sin took advantage of those commands and deceived me; it used the commands to kill me.*

12 *But still, the law itself is holy, and its commands are holy and right and good.*

13 *But how can that be? Did the law, which is good, cause my death? Of course not! Sin used what was good to bring about my condemnation to death. So we can see how terrible sin really is. It uses God's good commands for its own evil purposes.*

Romans 7:7-13

The willful failure of submission to God's Grace is Satan's malignant narcissism!

As you can now see, you need to be able to hold these seemingly diametrically opposed concepts of knowledge and faith in your mind at the same time. It is important to understand and respect these two powers – your sinful human evil desires and God's redeeming power that can save you from yourself. Your Ego-self does not want to give up control and become vulnerable to faith.

> *"The mark of a true genius is the ability to hold two seemingly contradictory ideas in mind at once."*
>
> Albert Einstein

The best minds are idiosyncratic and unpredictable as they follow the course of self-discovery. True intelligence is accepting that truth is deeper than what we can see and what our minds can comprehend.

Letting go of your mind, your ego and your earthly logic, leaves you with only few things left to hold onto ***Faith/Hope/Love***; that's what His Kingdom here is based on. God has predestined us who have made this choice to answer the spiritual pull of heaven to be like Him. You will be transformed to the likeness of God if you let go of protecting your Ego-self. Heaven will be one big supernatural Core. We will be part of God's Core. It will be the pure light of Truth. We will become pure with God; we will become part of His perfect Core forever.

Failure & Faith Summary Points

- We can accuse those that we have emotionally beaten down over time by using the power of scapegoating; blaming them for our own Core problems, leaving them lacking the emotional power to escape from the relationship. This is just like what Satan does to us, keeping us from God's redeeming grace. So by displacing our Core problems with blaming others, the Ego-Self does not have to face our own Core issues.

- Evil is defined as the use of power to destroy the spiritual growth of others for the sole purpose of defending and preserving their own narcissistic illness. People who hold on to this evil position deny the suffering of their guilt.

- Just like an air conditioner or refrigerator removes heat for cold to exist. So you can't make cold: it only exists when heat is not there. Similarly you can't make darkness; you must remove light for darkness to exist. Whenever and wherever God removes His Spirit, evil will exist. So God does not do evil, but He has created the space for it to exist by removing His Spirit. This process that God created gave His creation choice during this realm of time; the effect is that most things He has created are subject to change.

- Romantic relationships, friendships, business success, etc. are just expressions of fulfillment. They are not fulfillment itself. Fulfillment is the state of expressing who you really are, being the right person at your Core. It's about being fully alive. It's a feeling of wholeness, satisfaction, peace, rightness and harmony with the Creator; that can only happen through Failure and Faith.

- Most religions don't teach you to "let go" of trying to please God by our own efforts. The truth is that you need to accept that you are a natural born sinner, before God's grace can do its divine purpose and rescue you. It is about a life on the other side of your Ego-self. The key is to accept in our heart and mind that it's OK to fail at God's tests; so we can humbly grow in faith and appreciate His powerful grace.

- You need to be able to hold these seemingly diametrically opposed concepts of knowledge and faith in your mind at the same time. It is important to understand and respect these two powers – your sinful human evil desires and God's redeeming power that can save you from yourself. Your Ego-self does not want to give up control and become vulnerable to faith.

- The best minds are idiosyncratic and unpredictable as they follow the course of self-discovery. True intelligence is accepting that truth is deeper than what we can see and what our minds can comprehend.

CHAPTER SEVEN

The Conclusion

Developing God's Nature

If you are at the point in your life where you feel you must make a choice to let go and you don't follow a process of connecting with God and finding your chosen path, you will go back to your old life the way it was for the sake of not losing your mind and to protect the Ego-self.

One unique part about this process that I find fascinating is that we start to develop God's nature. I guess the more you hang around with somebody you start to look and behave more like them to others. These are the traits that will develop in your life if you follow this process and spend more time with Him each day. If you make this choice, you are predestined to become more: *Kind*, *Patient*, *Caring*, and *Sensitive* to spiritual things. People will look to you as a holder of the *Truth*, a *Teacher* of God's ways to the spiritually hungry and a beholder of the ability to *Love* and *Give* of yourself unconditionally. *Forgiver* of people making bad choices that hurt others. *Councilor* to heavy hearts. *Light* in this dark world, exposing the True-Self in others and *Revealing* the future Path of things to come, so others start to develop *Faith* and

Trust in God's perfect control. Being *Hopeful* in all things good and a sense of *Peace,* because God is in control of all outcomes, and I mean all outcomes!

> *For our earthly fathers disciplined us for a few years, doing the best they knew how. But God's discipline is always good for us, so that we might share in his holiness. No discipline is enjoyable while it is happening—it's painful! But afterward there will be a peaceful harvest of right living for those who are trained in this way. So take a new grip with your tired hands and strengthen your weak knees. Mark out a straight path for your feet so that those who are weak and lame will not fall but become strong.*
>
> Hebrews 12:10-13

God through the power of the Holy Spirit using Love & Grace is the only force that can melt cold hardened hearts of men and women. When His Spirit passes by our cold hardened hearts we can feel the warmth and even take in some of the heat that will last for a while, until the cold world cools our metal like hearts again.

The longer His warm Spirit is held next to our cold metal-like hearts, the more of His heat we take in. When we humble ourselves to Him and trust in His sacrifice to cover our sinful nature, praising and respectfully obeying Him for whom He really is. That is accepting at our Core that He is the King of Kings, Lord of Lords, Creator of all things and all powers. Then yielding our ego-selves, by letting down the prideful shields that seemingly protect us from His judgment, we find ourselves appreciating His unselfish sacrifice. It is critical to come to the realization of the truth that He is holding us up, not us holding Him up against this cold world. Only then, will we allow our cold and pride filled hearts to be in contact with His warm Spirit long enough to melt our hearts and let the spiritual Core healing work in us begin.

This is when His Spirit and our spirit start to become one!

It is just like the word *cleave* in the marriage covenant with God. In Genesis 2:24 the scriptures refer to becoming one flesh: or "Cleave," The Hebrew word here is "debaq" which means to make a permanent alliance with. In its noun form, the word refers to welding two pieces of metal together through the heat of the Holy Spirit. Some theologians have suggested that this term refers to a permanent action from God that cannot be undone.

In the same way when we humble ourselves before God and accept His sacrifice of His only begotten Son as our sacrificial atonement for our sins, the Holy Spirit melts into our cold hearts and welds Himself into us, becoming one with us and us with Him. This is the covenant that He promises to have with anyone that is willing to allow His warm, comforting and unconditional loving Spirit to come in contact with our cold hardened hearts.

Christians and unbelievers

As we walk through this cold world, Christ's Spirit should be flowing through us, touching cold-hardened hearts each day by giving off a high level spiritual energy signal that other hearts can feel. Their cold-hardened hearts will take in the heat from our spiritually-warmed hearts as we spend short segments of time with others.

When the Spirit of the living God holds a hard cold disobedient heart up against a humbly melted heart, over time that cold hard heart will begin to melt and allow God's restoration process to start! After softening, just like a welding process, that weld will become one new stronger metal if that heart chooses to allow the process to continue. If that cold hardened heart is not in contact long enough to melt and their ego won't relinquish control, they will rationally break the connection stopping the spiritual welding process with their Spirit. If that welding process is completed, it cannot be broken. That new heart at our Core is actually stronger than the original Core before the process began.

Christians and other Christians

God melts our hearts and welds us together with other Christians. Jesus said, "What you do to the least of them, you do to Me!" So if you as a Christian believe you are treating Jesus fairly, but are condescending to other Christians, it flows through back to God, because we are welded in spirit through the Holy Spirit.

For this reason we need to fellowship together and spend enough time with other Christians to have the heat of the Holy Spirit flowing through us to other hearts, welding us together and making that bond last for eternity.

Evidence You Are on the Right Path

These are the fruits that will show up from being on the right path:

1. Joy
2. Faith
3. Hope
4. Love
5. Peace

Joy

Joy is not searching for Love, Pleasure, Happiness, Peace or Comfort. Joy is being at peace with yourself and God. Joy is finding your chosen right Path for your life while feeling that you are fulfilling your Life Purpose. Knowing that you are called by the creator to stay on your Path for the blessing it will bring to others, and the blessings that make you so enviably happy that others will want a relationship with God just like you have.

Joy is when you know someone loves you unconditionally like God loves us the way a parent loves their child. Joy is finding that one person in this big world that loves you just the way you are. Joy also loves others unconditionally not needing any acceptance back in return to feed our Ego Self.

Faith

If you are Faithful you start bearing good fruit for yourself. We were raised to believe that unfaithfulness hurts others more than ourselves. But that is not true. It hurts our Ego Selves and our True Selves deep in our Cores. We cannot love ourselves and then truly love others if we are not honestly Faithful to our True Selves at our Core. Having a clear conscience by living a life of truth telling and Faithfulness, allows us to start respecting ourselves again; which is the foundation to loving ourselves. As in chapter six, until we give up on our Ego-Self through failure of trying to control our Path, we don't have real Faith in God; just in ourselves. God is Faithful whether or not we are Faithful to Him. We should be Faithful in all things and to all others in our lives. It is critical for a healthy Core and Path.

When we have that simple Faith in trusting His loving guidance without questioning, "God where are you taking me?" instead of praying for Him to do what we think He should do. That's when we have real Faith! Where two or more are gathered in His name with this kind of Faith, God can have a powerful effect in this evil world. This is a God-like experience that our brains can't comprehend. That's why we need to "Let go" or "yield" to God to make this Faith connection.

This scripture basically says anything that is not done in faith is a sin

Your personal convictions on such matters--exercise [them] as in God's presence, keeping them to yourself striving only to know the truth and obey His will. Blessed (happy, to be envied) is he who has no reason to judge himself for what he approves.

But the man who has doubts (uneasy conscience) about eating, and then eats, stands condemned before God, because he is not true to his convictions and he does not act from Faith. For whatever does not originate and proceed from Faith is sin [whatever is done without a conviction of its approval by God is sinful].

Romans 14:22-23

Hope

The greatest gift that God gives you during this time of transformation of your soul is *Hope!* When God takes the role of the Father in your life on a daily bases, you have a sense of security and peace so hope springs up in everything you think and do. God is the source of Hope!

Hope is a powerful tool in this world affected by time. It can give you peace and security in your heart and mind. If you let go of trying to control the outcomes in your life and just trust God to guide your Path, holding Him to His promise that all things work out for the good, for those that are called by the Spirit of God according to His purpose. God is the source of Hope!

Having Hope gives you courage to face adversity

Hope helps you feel protected and allows you to rest in a safe emotional place, even if the world is falling apart all around you. Just like the book of Job in the bible; the word *HOPE* is used over twenty times. Job used it as a tool to hang on to his faith, as God allowed Satan to destroy Job and the world around him.

Let all that I am wait quietly before God, for my Hope is in him.

Psalm 62:5

It seems so tragic that everyone under the sun suffers the same fate. That is why people are not more careful to be good. Instead, they choose their own mad course, for they have no Hope. There is nothing ahead but death anyway.

Ecclesiastes 9:3

Such things were written in the Scriptures long ago to teach us. And the Scriptures give us Hope and Encouragement as we wait patiently for God's promises to be fulfilled.

Romans 15:4

I pray that God, the Source of Hope, will fill you completely with joy and peace because you trust in him. Then you will overflow with confident Hope through the power of the Holy Spirit.

Romans 15:13

Faith is the confidence that what we Hope for will actually happen; it gives us assurance about things we cannot see.

Hebrews 11:1

Hope is what Faith is based on and it is the only thing that can please God. He wants us to hold Him to His promises and have *Hope* in the things to come.

Love

The evidence of *Love* will show up as a direct open honest intimacy with others in Christ. By this I mean a pure childlike approach, an unconditional appreciation of the intimate connection founded in *Love*. What ends up happening when *Love* is there, truth is emitted. It allows truth to be the foundation of the relationship. Without unselfish *Love*, truth cannot be sustained.

You can't sustain Love without truth and you can't sustain truth without Love.

There are some people who are communicating the truth, but because if is not done in *Love*, it will not be accepted in people's hearts and minds. If people try to express *Love* not being based in truth, it's not unconditional *Love* that can only come from God. Our *Love* comes from a root of ego driven desire and will not bare good lasting fruit.

Most of the time *Love* is an ego driven desire for acceptance. It's narcissistic medicine for the ego. True *Love* or *Love* founded in truth comes from your True Self, not your Ego Self or your insecure mind. That's why when you are feeling an intimate connection of the heart that the mind is trying to understand, you are experiencing that true honest *Love* connection that can only come from God. It is not physical or just emotional, but rather a spiritual connection of God's *Love* flowing back and forth between two beings that have Christ at their Cores. It's not a gift to the other party from you but a gift *"through you"* from God. You can only be a vessel of His *Love*. All pure unconditional *Love* comes from God. We have no capacity to generate this on our own. Unconditional *Love*, Agape-*Love* cannot be earned or created by mankind. *True Love expects nothing in return!*

Wherever there is Love there is healing; it is a fruit of Love.

16 *I pray that from His glorious, unlimited resources He will empower you with inner strength through His Spirit.*

17 *Then Christ will make His home in your hearts as you trust in Him. Your roots will grow down into God's Love and keep you strong.*

18 *And may you have the power to understand, as all God's people should, how wide, how long, how high, and how deep His Love is.*

19 *May you experience the Love of Christ, though it is too great to understand fully! Then you will be made complete with all the fullness of life and power that comes from God.*

Ephesians 3:16-19

Peace

What does it mean to have peace that passes all understanding? The Jews were chosen to seek the truth with their minds while desiring Peace in their hearts. They were given wisdom, knowledge and the Mosaic Law. That chosen Path did not set them free from themselves, or allow them to let go by the power of Abraham's faith.

By rejecting the Messiah and holding onto the Law for self-worth in God's eyes and power over each other in their culture, they have never experienced the peace that comes from being forgiven through Grace alone. Instead it consumed them in a state of ego driven debate, using the detail of the Law to judge their level of righteousness between each other, other cultures and their personal relationship with God.

This Path of Do's & Don'ts never leads to true Peace, but to a feeling deep inside of always falling short of being accepted by a perfect God. This position keeps them from finding that Peace that's beyond understanding. That Peace is only found by being forgiven through a childlike faith of trusting in a merciful God that will transform at the Core. All you have to do is accept the truth about how sinful you really are and stop protecting yourself from Him.

The most wonderful fruit that shows up after a transformation directed by God, is this Peace you feel when you enter into His Divine presence. It is something that you can't seem to figure out with your mind but it is just there any time you desire it. Many humans seek this peace by trying to control their minds through Eastern religions. Most of them use processes to try and control the mind like Yoga, meditation, seclusion, and even drugs. Most ancient native Indian cultures around the world used drugs to find a peace on the other side of self; just like so many young people today. All of these processes to find Peace have little residual compared to the lasting Peace of God's Grace.

Many people today seek truth from the Internet to find peace of mind just like the tower of Babel years ago, where humans built a tall structure dedicated to knowledge, trying to find

God's wisdom. Just like so many religions of today. True Peace is not achieved by spiritual work through knowledge or worldly sacrifice, but by letting go and trusting in God's redeeming Grace alone.

Peace is an emotional fruit that comes from the gift of eternal life.

What Fruit is coming from your Core?

I believe the most inclusive critical guiderail; would be having God Divinely guiding your True Self in lieu of being guided by your Ego-self. Here are some examples of behaviors that reveal which one is stronger at your Core at this time.

God-Centered

Humble, Thankful, Merciful, Patient, Trusting, Just, Selfless, Transparent, Truthful, Kind, Loving, Hopeful, Sensitive, Broken, Weak, Open & Honest and Future Confident

Self-Centered

Justified, Strong, Defensive, Controlling, Impatient, Desperate, Proud, Victimized, Blaming, Positioning and Worried about the Future

Counter-intuitive

The hardest thing to accept with our developed minds is that most revelations of truth are counter-intuitive to the way we think. So the more logical we are, the harder it is to accept this counter-intuitive part of Faith that bridges the gap between knowledge and truth.

Here are some examples of the concluding perspective on counter-intuitive thoughts in this book.

- Dying to yourself to find your way.
- You have to lose your life to gain it.
- If you hold on too tight you will lose it, whatever it is.
- You have to "let go" to receive what is good and right for you.

The bible gives us a series of counter-intuitive concepts in the Beatitudes. We just have to understand them in our hearts and minds while we trust God to prove them out in our lives.

Evidence of a Divine Relationship

Having a relationship with God can be more challenging and confusing, but working to meet God's Law will never give you the answers to the deep questions of the heart. Religion is about humans defining God to justify their self-desired Core and Path. Relationship with God is about our transformational process of the Core and faith in God to reveal our Path. That's the evidence of a healthy Divine relationship.

Having a relationship with God is critical for the light of truth and the companionship of God the Father on your Path.

If we have a dependent relationship with the Father God it is foolish to make plans or worry about our future. He has everything under control in our lives: our health, our relationships, our financial security, our peace and safety. God is the ultimate planner and controller. If He is for us, who can be against us? It is easy to have faith in God and our future if we just accept everything above as logical facts of truth. Then we will live happy and blessed lives that others will desire, realizing that true peace is there on the other side of self, if they also "let go" of control and start trusting God fully.

Having an open and honest relationship with God gives you joy and comfort when you understand the unique role of the trinity and the relationships with your Core and Path. When you start to trust Him with every aspect of your life, the fruit of comfort that you have in Him is joy. If you try to please Him with your efforts you will always fall short. This brings you back to the edge needing to be rescued again through Grace; keeping your Ego-Self in check.

Recognizable Conditions

Recognizable conditions are not activities; they are reflections of a state of being. These conditions should be recognizable in each Life Ring. They should be emanating from your Core, which would confirm in your heart and mind that you are on the right Path and aligned with your Life Purpose.

These conditions are NOT future outcomes, objectives, acquired assets or quantitative goals. Even though, that's what your Ego self would naturally think. Achieved milestones are not healthy recognizable conditions for your True Self. The real recognizable conditions are being aligned with your Core and bring a state of peace and saneness to your heart and mind. You will have a clear conscience knowing you are being true to yourself and are being on purpose in your life.

Worry: the Cancer of Faith

One condition you will recognize in a faith based life is that you won't be worrying as much about outcomes in your life like you use too. Others will notice the difference in you that you are calmer about issues and outcomes that others are worrying about. Worry is a natural human emotion for survival. It is linked to time. Without time, there is no need for worry, because nothing changes. Being confined to time makes it hard to see time having an end. You can worry about the past and you can worry about the present. But most of the time we worry about the future, even if it is the next second.

If you worry about the future it is normally based in fear or doubt. But if you have real faith, you don't worry about anything. True faith will replace worry by trusting God to control future outcomes. If not you will only have faith in yourself to control the future, trying to protect yourself or someone you care about. One of the most ironic behaviors I believe is when people ask God in prayer to help control the future for what they are worrying about at that time. The Holy Spirit can prod us to pray for things in the future so when they happen, it builds our faith in God control.

Another analogy is a child asking their parent for things. A child could be worried about outcomes at school or in their social life. Or as simple as saying things to their parents like "When will this or that happen?" It's like you saying, "God, I want you to control the future the way I want it to turn out." God already knows the future. So what are we doing worrying about anything that's going to happen in the future? We can't control the outcome anyway. All we show God when we worry is that we have no faith in Him.

Worry only comes from your Ego Self for self-protection. This could be worrying about anything, from a pimple on your face to worrying about the end of the world. Even terrorism is not about the attack, but the *worry* of an attack happening in the future. The Muslim Jihād movement focuses on creating worry and fear in the hearts of Christians. They don't see us as God fearing. They see us as Muslim fearing and future fearing infidels. If we have real faith in God, there is *nothing* to fear. You won't fear tomorrow or any day in the future. You won't fear the deception of Satan's power to control outcomes outside God's plan. You won't even fear the sting of death itself. You will only fear God. He is the only one in control. There is no power controlling the future, except God!

> *"Dear friends, don't be afraid of those who want to kill your body; they cannot do any more to you after that. But I'll tell you whom to fear. Fear God, who has the power to kill you and then throw you into hell. Yes, He's the one to fear.*
>
> Luke 12:4-5

Reciprocal Relationships

Another interesting condition you will recognize is that God will bring people into your life to help you stay on your Path and at the same time you will help them in what they are going through in their life at that time. Having relationships in your life that are balanced in exchange of resources from spiritual to temporal is critical for your growth of your True Self. The resentful givers, narcissistic takers and insecure relationships in your life will slowly move out of your day-to-day life. This also is essential for discovering and developing a balanced Core and Path.

There is a book written by Melissa Giovagnoli that covers this subject in more detail. *The Nanosecond Networlders: Changing Lives in An Instant Forever - A Modern Business Fairytale* is available on Amazon.

Emotional Needs

One example of a recognizable condition is some of these basic emotional needs will start to be fulfilled from the people in your life that you love. As God starts to transform your Core, you start to care about these needs in others. You will be pleasantly surprised to find you receive what you give out. Here are some basic human emotional needs in an alphabetical list with no ranking of importance. Although you might want to rank these for yourself to get a better look at your current emotional needs.

- ***Admiration***
- ***Affection***
- ***Appreciation***
- ***Commitment***
- ***Financial needs***
- ***Open & Honest Conversation***
- ***Physical Attractiveness***
- ***Recreational Companionship***
- ***Respect***
- ***Sexual Fulfillment***
- ***Trust***

Future Revealed

God loves to reveal the future to those that let go and have faith in Him. He loves to tell us what the future holds because He is the only one who knows it. He is not affected by time; so He can see the future and the past at the same time. This is what separates the living God from all other gods. God created the future before the past began and He loves to reveal our paths to us as any good father would here on earth at the right time to help guide us on our Path.

Everything has already been decided. It was known long ago what each person would be. So there's no use arguing with God about your destiny.

Ecclesiastes 6:10

1 *"I have told you these things so that you won't abandon your faith.*

2 *For you will be expelled from the synagogues, and the time is coming when those who kill you will think they are doing a holy service for God.*

3 *This is because they have never known the Father or me.*

4 *Yes, I'm telling you these things now, so that when they happen, you will remember my warning. I didn't tell you earlier because I was going to be with you for a while longer.*

John 16:1-4

Jesus loved to reveal the future events to His followers every chance He could, because is He had God's nature, because He was God. God is the Core and Path of all creation. He is the "I am." Because we are created in *His* image, we never feel fulfilled following our Core and Path, until we let go and find the peace and comfort of being aligned with His Core and Path.

You are predestined to be saved from your Ego-Self if you receive into your Core the Living Spirit of the Son of God. This will continue for the rest of your life. For God to each you through failure, your Ego-Self will make every effort to regain control of your life again as your life returns back to normal. Staying on purpose is critical to not going back.

Rescuing others

Now that God has rescued us from ourselves, we are called by His Spirit to help those that are oppressed by sin. We are rescuing them from their own life damaging sinful selves and also the oppressing evil abuse that this world and others have used to control them. This is the Kingdom work of God's Spirit in this world filled with sin.

Summary

One of the keys to appreciating who God really is, is through comprehending how seriously He takes one-on-one relationships with His creations. That is the most important trait we have in our make-up from being created in His image. The key to a happy, peace filled life is staying aligned with the *Idiosyncratic Core & Path* that God has planned for you. Accepting that your *True Self* deep in your Core is where you will find the Truth and the Light to reveal your *Path* is the counter-intuitive key to a balanced life of faith and peace.

Knowledge can feed your Ego and the Internet is like the "Tree of Knowledge." It feeds our minds with thoughts and desires. It is just the like the *"Apple"* that Eve took a bite of that awakened the Ego. The Bible says that just before man figures out the secret of life itself, the end will come. We are created in God's image with an ego and power to choose to live for ourselves or die to ourselves. We have the choice to become our own god or give up the power God gave us, to *"let go"* and allow Him be the Master of our souls. It's our choice!

Knowledge from that tree started expanding from the beginning of time and has now become the source of truth for seekers of knowledge as we enter into the end of this age. Information allows people to make choices about relationships based on what they think and not what they feel in their hearts. That is why so many people are getting divorced today. Love, in a knowledge-based culture is conditional, when God wants us to love like Him: unconditionally. Knowledge puffs up the ego and justifies scapegoating our problems that we create for ourselves onto others.

As knowledge changes from a scarce resource to an overwhelming flood of information, it becomes easier to judge others and condemn them, so we feel better about ourselves. Kindness and unconditional love will be the only powers that will keep people faithful in relationships. Who would have ever thought that the tree of knowledge in the Garden of Eden would grow into this flood of information we now call the Internet. It creates a hunger for more and more information in almost every human brain. When the real truth is counter-intuitive to the way we think, it only makes it harder to get to the True Self deep in our Core.

I now know that I am not where I need to be in my transformation to being like Christ, but I am glad that I am not where I was before this all started.

Follow God not others!

Following a leader is easier than leading your own life. Because there is no need for agonizing over complex decisions, planning future outcomes, exercising initiative, risk of being unpopular, or exert much courage. The role of a blind follower is the role of a trusting child in a controlling relationship. Psychologically you become dependent on the leader by handing over your power of choice, just as a child's relationship with a parent. The individual adult is the captain of his or her own ship and is responsible for their Path through choice.

This process provides the keys to discovering your True Self. You are not the Creator of your Path. This hidden treasure is found through a spiritual connection with God and a simple step of faith. That's why it has to be counter-intuitive to the mind.

> *I pray that from His glorious, unlimited resources He will empower you with inner strength through His Spirit. Then Christ will make His home in your hearts as you trust in Him. Your roots will grow down into God's love and keep you strong. And may you have the power to understand, as all God's people should, how wide, how long, how high, and how deep His love is. May you experience the love of Christ, though it might be too great to understand fully. Then you will be made complete with all the fullness of life and power that comes from God.*
>
> Ephesians 3:16-19

May your conscience testify that you have conducted yourself in the world in obedience and honesty that come from God, not in human wisdom, but in the grace of God especially in your relationship with others!

Jesus, unlike the founders or prophets of any other major religion, holds out hope for every human to be reconciled to the Creator God.

There is no greater joy in this life then to have God pursue you to "let go" of the cares of this world and live a life of faith, enjoying what God has planned to bring in your Path each day.

I now know that I am not where I need to be in my transformation to being like Christ, but I am glad that I am not where I was before this all started.

In final conclusion I want to humbly thank you for giving me the time to share what I believe is truth that is essential for spiritually surviving in these dark times.

APPENDIX

Concentric Life Rings

These Rings are strongly interrelated, but need a clear separation from each other while being bridged by your Life Purpose.

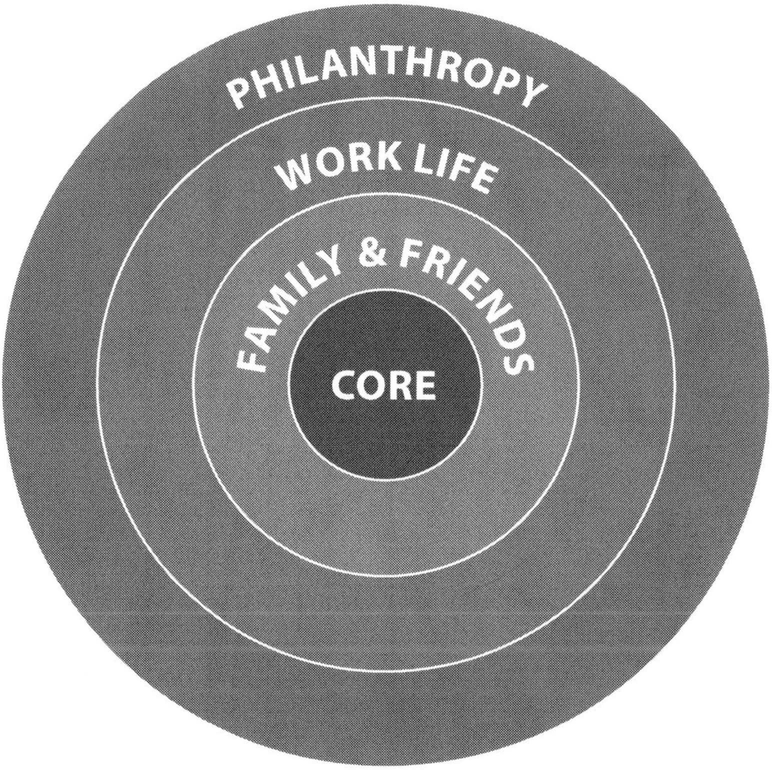

From Concentric Life Rings in Chapter One

Dialectic Approach to Planning

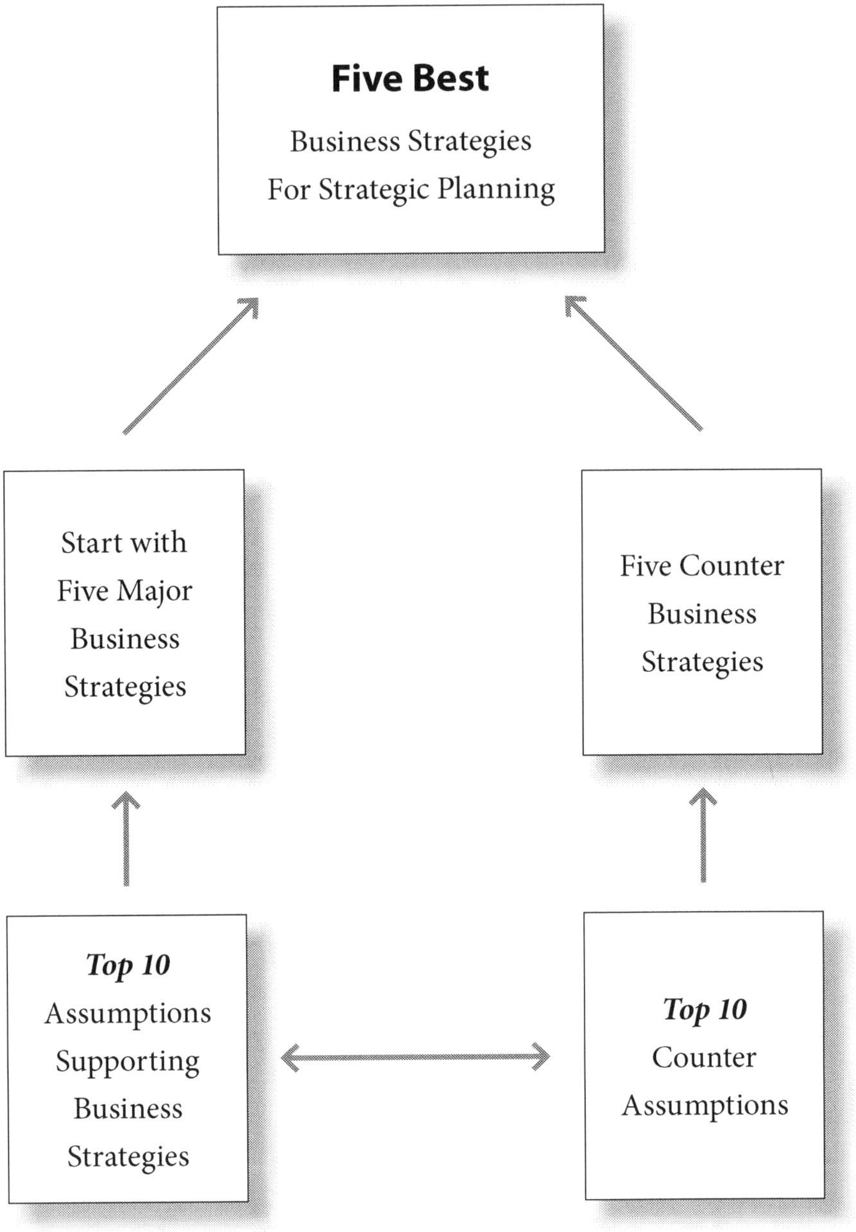

From Work Life Ring in Chapter One

Psalm 103

1 Let all that I am praise the Lord; with my whole heart, I will praise His holy name.

2 Let all that I am praise the Lord; may I never forget the good things He does for me.

3 He forgives all my sins and heals all my diseases.

4 He redeems me from death and crowns me with love and tender mercies.

5 He fills my life with good things. My youth is renewed like the eagles!

6 The Lord gives righteousness and justice to all who are treated unfairly.

7 He revealed His character to Moses and his deeds to the people of Israel.

8 The Lord is compassionate and merciful, slow to get angry and filled with unfailing love.

9 He will not constantly accuse us, nor remain angry forever.

10 He does not punish us for all our sins; He does not deal harshly with us, as we deserve.

11 For His unfailing love toward those who fear Him is as great as the height of the heavens above the earth.

12 He has removed our sins as far from us as the east is from the west.

13 *The Lord is like a father to His children, tender and compassionate to those who fear Him.*

14 *For He knows how weak we are; He remembers we are only dust.*

15 *Our days on earth are like grass; like wildflowers, we bloom and die.*

16 *The wind blows, and we are gone—as though we had never been here.*

17 *But the love of the Lord remains forever with those who fear Him. His salvation extends to the children's children*

18 *of those who are faithful to His covenant, of those who obey His commandments!*

19 *The Lord has made the heavens His throne; from there He rules over everything.*

20 *Praise the Lord, you angels, you mighty ones who carry out His plans, listening for each of His commands.*

21 *Yes, praise the Lord, you armies of angels who serve Him and do His will!*

22 *Praise the Lord, everything He has created, everything in all His kingdom.*

Let all that I am praise the Lord.

ABOUT THE AUTHOR

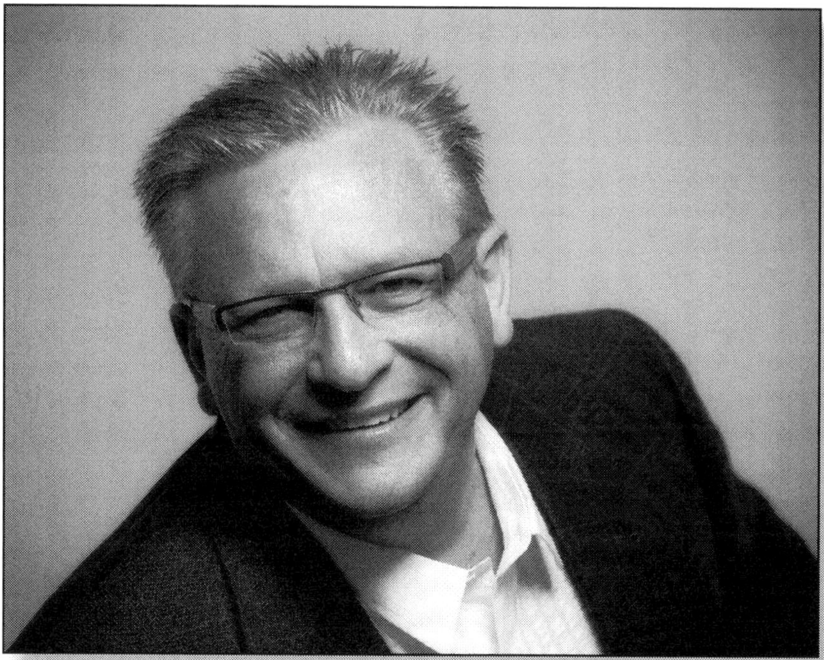

Paul Omdoll was the Chief Business Development Officer of The Colman Group, Inc. which included both San Jamar and Chef Revival brands. From 1984 to 2011 Paul positioned the company as the industry leader in hospitality products for the Food Service and JanSan markets, taking sales from $1 million to over $80 million. In February of 2012, Paul and his partner sold their interests in SJCR and is currently the Executive Senior Vice President of Strategic Development for the new commercial company. After a stress-induced stroke, a goodwill trip to Africa and a divorce, he was compelled to write his first book.

In his spare time, Paul enjoys international travel, flying small aircrafts, scuba diving, golf, tennis, biking, boating, downhill skiing and Harley riding. He has two adult children and three grandchildren. Paul now lives in Naples, Florida.

For a more in-depth bio and a link to his blog to stay connected, please visit www.coreandpath.com

Made in United States
Orlando, FL
14 June 2022

18799537R00130